Theology and Medicine in Conversation

Theology and Medicine in Conversation

How the Healing Happens

Benjamin R. Doolittle and
S. Mark Heim

t&tclark
LONDON · NEW YORK · OXFORD · NEW DELHI · SYDNEY

T&T CLARK

Bloomsbury Publishing Plc, 50 Bedford Square, London, WC1B 3DP, UK
Bloomsbury Publishing Inc, 1359 Broadway, New York, NY 10018, USA
Bloomsbury Publishing Ireland, 29 Earlsfort Terrace, Dublin 2, D02 AY28, Ireland

BLOOMSBURY, T&T CLARK and the T&T Clark logo are trademarks
of Bloomsbury Publishing Plc

First published in Great Britain 2026

Copyright © Benjamin R. Doolittle and S. Mark Heim, 2026

Benjamin R. Doolittle and S. Mark Heim have asserted their right under the Copyright,
Designs and Patents Act, 1988, to be identified as Author of this work.

For legal purposes the Acknowledgements on pp. xiii-xiv constitute an extension
of this copyright page.

Cover design: Elena Durey
Cover image: The Blind man of Jericho 1650 Nicolas Poussin 1594-1665
© Peter Horree/Alamy

All rights reserved. No part of this publication may be: i) reproduced or transmitted in
any form, electronic or mechanical, including photocopying, recording or by means of
any information storage or retrieval system without prior permission in writing from
the publishers; or ii) used or reproduced in any way for the training, development or
operation of artificial intelligence (AI) technologies, including generative AI technologies.
The rights holders expressly reserve this publication from the text and data mining
exception as per Article 4(3) of the Digital Single Market Directive (EU) 2019/790.

Bloomsbury Publishing Plc does not have any control over, or responsibility for, any third-
party websites referred to or in this book. All internet addresses given in this book were
correct at the time of going to press. The author and publisher regret any inconvenience
caused if addresses have changed or sites have ceased to exist, but can accept no
responsibility for any such changes.

Library of Congress Control Number: 2025943453

ISBN: HB: 978-0-5677-1536-4
PB: 978-0-5677-1535-7
ePDF: 978-0-5677-1538-8
eBook: 978-0-5677-1537-1

Typeset by Deanta Global Publishing Services, Chennai, India
Printed and bound in Great Britain

For product safety related questions contact productsafety@bloomsbury.com.

To find out more about our authors and books visit www.bloomsbury.com
and sign up for our newsletters.

Contents

Preface vii
Acknowledgments xiii

1 **Better Together: Two Paths for Healing** 1

2 **The Wound of Mortality: Theology and Medicine in the Anatomy Lab** 17

3 **The Ages of Medicine and Faith** 35

4 **Pain, Prayer, and Placebo** 67

5 **Healing at the End** 89

6 **Is Religion Good For You?** 107

7 **Faith and Contagion in the Public Square** 131

8 **Stigma and Health: The HIV Epidemic** 149

9 **Addiction: Therapy of Hope and Forgiveness** 167

10 **Burnout as Spiritual Crisis** 183

11 **Cancer, Immortality, and Christology: The Theological Resonance of Henrietta Lacks** 203

Epilogue 219
Index 229

Preface

Why is a book like this needed? The time is ripe to revisit the relations between medicine and religion, and particularly to explore their positive interaction. There are at least three reasons to clarify this argument at this moment.

The first is that individual doctors, pastors, chaplains, and above all patients (a category that eventually includes all of us) often find estrangement or assumed conflicts between religion and medicine causing harm and frustrating healing. Many others in the health care domain do not register the mutual influences of the two as important clinical and pastoral considerations, regardless of whether that interaction figures prominently in their own experience.

Second, a new academic field studying the relation of religion and medicine has grown up over the last fifty years.[1] That academic work is little known or appreciated outside a small circle, but its implications are broad and significant. Our claim that medicine and religion belong together draws deeply on this research and aims to share it more widely.

Third, both of the authors of this book are teachers, and we see this connection as an educational and professional imperative. Theological education pays little attention to the medical arena except as the setting for pastoral care, and medical education has paid little attention to spiritual resources—although this is changing in many medical schools. This book seeks to expand and encourage an open conversation between the two educational settings in which the authors are rooted.

Cross-disciplinary interaction is often stalled at the start, especially among academics, by the fact that those well trained in one area are hesitant to stray into another where they are not. One of us, Ben Doolittle, is among the rare people with full standing in both areas: a physician and professor at Yale Medical School and an ordained pastor in the Reformed Church in

---

[1] This new phase dates from the pioneering work of Dr. David Larson and others in the 1970s. See David B. Larson, Jeffrey S. Levin, and Harold G. Koenig, *Faith, Medicine, and Science: A Festschrift in Honor of Dr. David B. Larson* (Binghamton, NY: Haworth Pastoral Press, 2005).

America serving a local congregation in New Haven. Both vocationally and personally, he has spent most of his life reflecting on these issues, leading to his co-founding of Yale's Program for Medicine, Spirituality, and Religion. Mark Heim is a theologian on the faculty at Yale Divinity School. He has been teaching about science and theology for many years, as well as writing extensively about Christianity and religious pluralism. His work at Andover Newton Seminary at Yale has been oriented toward preparing those who become pastors and chaplains, whose ministry necessarily involves constant practical encounter with illness and death.

Ben and Mark met serendipitously in 2016 when Mark had recently arrived as part of Andover Newton Theological School's relocation from Boston to become part of Yale Divinity School. What began as a fascinating conversation quickly turned into both a stimulating friendship and a popular course on theology and medicine. In addition to theological students, the course attracts participants from across the university. These include students from the undergraduate campus, the nursing school, the school of public health, the school of management, and the business school, as well as auditors from various parts of the medical school. Our class meetings purposely alternate between physical locations at the medical school and at the divinity school, two different kinds of educational home "turf."

Students often come with a story of their own engagement with the medical system. A loved one tragically died. They themselves endured a chronic illness or experienced a dramatic recovery. As ministers or as health care providers, they have grappled with the mysteries of healing and suffering. Some of the students aspire to chaplaincy or to doctoral programs in medical research or ethics. They bring a keen interest in the intersection of theology and medicine because that is where pain and dilemmas are often found, as well as healing and hope.

Most of the creativity we see emerge in and around our classroom has little to do with us, and everything to do with the unusual space it offers for exploration. Our topic lies closely adjacent to many others, but its value stems from its sprawl across disciplinary expectations and its suspension of mutual suspicions that isolate these areas. The contents of this book, and indeed the idea for the book itself, were both born from the joy and curiosity we experienced in conversation, in the classroom, and in the community of a widening circle of graduates. We have tried to write with a united outlook, but the book clearly reflects two different voices, and some vignettes are solely Mark's or Ben's. For example, in Chapter 8 the clinical vignette of caring for Rosa is from Ben's practice. We let these stories stand on their own, reflective of our shared work, to highlight the themes of each chapter. We realize that the eclectic character of this discussion is not attractive to all, including some of our academic peers. We may try to be a little bit of everything to everybody. In that, we certainly fail. But we hope to provide enough sparks to make the conversation richer and deeper.

This book is not a historical survey of medicine and religion, of which one may find outstanding examples in the works of Gary Ferngren and Jeff Levin.[2] It is not an encyclopedic survey of research in this area, for which one may turn to Harold Koenigs' landmark compendium *Handbook on Religion and Health*.[3] This is not a book about pastoral care, chaplaincy, or biomedical ethics, although we touch on the content of those fields, and believe the broad issues we address are helpful for those at the bedside in various capacities. Our book does not address the profound questions about the structure of our health care system, which have deep religious and moral dimensions. But we feel confident that the harmony of spiritual and biological perspectives we commend will be one aspect of a health care system with both optimal medical outcomes and high levels of trust. What this book offers relates to what the portion of its title *"in conversation"* suggests. Each chapter intends to share a spark of conversation between theology and medicine that we have found stimulating and provocative for our students and for ourselves.

There are obvious limitations to our outlooks. We both come from Protestant Christian perspectives. Mark is an American Baptist minister and seminary professor with decades of teaching and church leadership. Ben is an internist, pediatrician, and ordained minister in the Reformed Church in America who teaches at Yale Medical School. We recognize that this conversation between theology and medicine is inherently skewed by our specific perspectives. We also recognize the rich legacy of healing from other cultures and perspectives. Mark, in particular, is a scholar in comparative or interreligious theology and has good reason to appreciate the depths of wisdom found particularly in the Buddhist traditions he has studied. We are not experts in the interface of medicine with other major traditions than our own. We fear our thoughts would ring hollow and would do a disservice to

---

[2] Jeffrey S. Levin, *Religion and Medicine: A History of the Encounter between Humanity's Two Greatest Institutions* (New York: Oxford University Press, 2020); Gary B. Ferngren, *Medicine and Religion: A Historical Introduction* (Baltimore, MD: Johns Hopkins University Press, 2014).
[3] Harold G. Koenig, Dana E. King, and Verna Benner Carson, *Handbook of Religion and Health*, 2nd ed. (Oxford; New York: Oxford University Press, 2012).

those rich traditions if we claimed to represent them. To avoid weak generality and to directly acknowledge this limitation, we center the dialogue between medicine and theology in our own Christian perspectives.[4]

We realize that Christian faith and Christian churches are currently declining as sociological features in American life, and that the realization of the promise for religious/medical harmony involves appreciation for a wide spectrum of religious traditions and emergent practices. This means that both religious caregivers, such as chaplains, and medical providers will be faced with an increasingly challenging spectrum of particulars. This book is thus just one contribution to that discussion. It seeks to support the integration we commend for individual Christians and Christian communities with medical institutions. And, since the medical institutions and culture around us are largely shaped by the Christian tradition, it seeks also to identify aspects of this history that may be of broader common value.

A Brief Outline

Chapter 1 articulates our basic thesis: medicine and religion belong together. We review what connects them and the forces that tend to pull them apart.

The first section of the book, Chapters 2 through 5, focuses on the grand themes that religion and medicine hold in common: mortality, pain, suffering, the process of dying. These are points at which the two perspectives tend to flow together, where it becomes hard to distinguish what is being "treated" in a medical sense from what is being interpreted and transformed in a religious sense. We start in Chapter 2 where modern medical education has traditionally begun, in the anatomy lab. We consider the nature of ministry and medicine as vocations, both rooted in the shared wound of mortality. In Chapter 3 we look back briefly at the historical context of this relationship, at the integration of faith and medicine in the past, the changing models of medical healing, and the resulting changes in the interface of religion with medicine. In Chapter 4 we consider pain and suffering, and the

---

[4] And even then, we cannot do justice to the full variety of approaches that exist across the Christian spectrum. On this variety, see Ronald L. Numbers and Darrel W. Amundsen, *Caring and Curing: Health and Medicine in the Western Religious Traditions* (Baltimore, MD: Johns Hopkins University Press, 1998).

spectrum across which neurological pain interacts with subjective suffering. In Chapter 5 we address the "lost art of dying," the arena of end of life care, where this dialogue has never been truly absent and where it is receiving more recognition and support.

Section Two, Chapters 6–10, turns to a number of more specific topics. We begin with Chapter 6, which addresses the particular statistical language of modern medicine. In an age of evidence based medicine, research has become a key driver of conversation between theology and medicine, and it comes up in almost all of our topics. The data on religion's effect on health, the breadth and depth of research on the relevance of religious practices for health outcomes, are not generally appreciated. But such research is key to the case for religion to be considered as an integral feature in clinical care, and not just the idiosyncratic concern of individual physicians and individual patients.

We then proceed to consider some specific medical case studies. Chapters 7 and 8 consider particular issues arising around contagious diseases and faith, reflecting on pandemics throughout history (including Covid) and then specifically on HIV. The next pair of chapters, Chapter 9 on addiction and Chapter 10 on burnout in clergy and medical workers, turn to topics where faith and treatment are actively entwined, and most particularly to one where spiritual and medical care givers figure prominently among the afflicted.

Finally, in Section Three, we turn to two concluding reflections. Chapter 11, "Cancer, Immortality, and Christology: The Theological Resonance of Henrietta Lacks," takes the extraordinary story of Henrietta Lacks and the role of her "immortal" cells as a lens through which to explore many of the themes we have raised throughout the book. The epilogue, "Last Things and First Things," links the religious category of "things made new" (eschatology) with the imminent expansion of medicine into the realm of human transformation.

Because the course we teach involves things like a trip to the anatomy lab, visits to the medical museum's "brain room," and discussion of medical conditions with which students may have painful immediate experience, our syllabus initially offered a "trigger warning" to alert people to these features and to advise them they could seek adjustments if needed to be sure the course was safe for them. One of our guest speakers chided us a bit for this approach. No meaningful learning experience is entirely "safe" in terms of its transformative possibilities, he said. Teachers should protect their students from danger, but not from the testing that can flower in growth. We have certainly seen that kind of growth. Several of our Divinity school students have gone on to enroll in nursing or medical school degrees. Some of the students with medical backgrounds have added theological study to their personal vocations or integrated religion into their visions of practice and research. One student modeled her career after a saint we discussed in class. Another has gone on to become an internationally recognized researcher in the field of pain and prayer. Several students have turned their final course projects and papers into publications in the peer reviewed literature. With each passing year, we hear how seeds planted in class discussions and projects have grown into subsequent forms of professional and vocational integration. We still give advance information to students about what may be troubling components of the class. But we also offer an additional trigger warning: this class might change your life. It has changed ours.

Acknowledgments

Any person whose care or treatment is mentioned in this book has given their permission and names and details have been changed to preserve anonymity, unless the person specifically approved their identification.

We are grateful for the many supporters who made this project possible. In particular, we are grateful for the Yale faculty and scholars who greatly enhance the energy of our course. Sarah Drummond, the dean of Andover Newton Seminary at Yale Divinity School, has given us administrative and personal support from the beginning. Every year Charles Duncan, Linda Honan, and Bill Stewart welcome the Divinity School students to the anatomy lab. More than that, they model compassion, wisdom and a generous spirit in that delicate, sacred space. In that same spirit, we convey our most heartfelt thanks to Melissa Grafe, the Director of the Cushing Historical Library at the Yale Medical School and Terry Dagradi, the Curator of the Cushing Center. They put on a terrific presentation—priceless historic manuscripts, moving patient photos, and a captivating museum display. More than sharing the resources of a great university collection, they inspire an infectious zeal and engaging kindness.

We are grateful also for those who have been guest lecturers in our course. Lydia Dugdale is a world expert in the lost art of dying. Gary Strichartz is one-of-a-kind: a researcher in pain and a hospital chaplain. Karina Danvers shares her journey with authenticity and openness, inspiring us all. Carolyn Roberts is doing path-breaking scholarship on race and medicine, in the past and in the present. Augustine Boetang fills the classroom with energy and insight in his conversation about race, religion, and science. Tyler VanderWeele shared his unparalleled statistical insights on the relevant research. Marta Illueca was already a pioneer in religion and medicine when she came to our class and her recent writings have enriched the field further. Michael Balboni helped orient and inspire us with his longstanding contributions in this area, when we were just getting started with our course. Debora Jackson recruited and shepherded a delightful continuing education cohort of pastors who followed our course and shared their experiences. Together, this gang make for a vibrant, engaging course which is such a joy.

We are grateful to the Templeton Foundation for the grant money that supported the continuing education program just mentioned, and to the Dialogue on Science, Ethics, and Religion of the American Academy for the Advancement of Science, which administered that grant. We express our appreciation to the Journal of the American Medical Association for permission to quote extensively in Chapter 1 from the John Stone poem originally published there. We want to thank Rona Gordon for her editorial insights and keen suggestions in the final stages of our manuscript.

Above all, we are grateful for the students who have taken the course over the years. Their wisdom, cheerfulness, and engagement has inspired and challenged us. The book is full of the contributions from those who have participated in our course and steadily added new fuel to the fire of conversation. We express our sincere thanks to every one of those students and collaborators, for each has left some mark on this project.

References

Ferngren, Gary B. *Medicine and Religion: A Historical Introduction*. Baltimore, MD: Johns Hopkins University Press, 2014.

Koenig, Harold G., Dana E. King, and Verna Benner Carson. *Handbook of Religion and Health*, 2nd ed. Oxford; New York: Oxford University Press, 2012.

Larson, David B., Jeffrey S. Levin, and Harold G. Koenig. *Faith, Medicine, and Science: A Festschrift in Honor of Dr. David B. Larson*. Binghamton, NY: Haworth Pastoral Press, 2005.

Levin, Jeffrey S. *Religion and Medicine: A History of the Encounter between Humanity's Two Greatest Institutions*. New York: Oxford University Press, 2020.

Numbers, Ronald L., and Darrel W. Amundsen. *Caring and Curing: Health and Medicine in the Western Religious Traditions*. Baltimore, MD: Johns Hopkins University Press, 1998.

1

Better Together
Two Paths for Healing

Chapter Outline

Medicine and Religion Belong Together	1
Positive Shared Elements	3
Challenges	6
Healthy Differences	8
Two Languages for Healing	9

Medicine and Religion Belong Together

Our thesis is simple. Medicine and religion belong together.[1] For almost all of human history they were deeply interwoven. In the modern world they are often seen at odds, or carefully isolated from each other. We do not believe this is either a *healthy* stance for medical practice or a *faithful* stance

---

[1] "Religion" is a much-debated word and may connote only organized religious bodies. We use the word much more broadly to include dispositions and practices regarding ultimate purpose and meaning, particularly beliefs and practices whose references are transrational or supranational. We speak explicitly as Christians, but for the purpose of our primary thesis—medicine and religion belong together—this Christian focus is illustrative, not exclusive. The ways in which various traditions or aspects of traditions might have comparably varying impacts on particular medical conditions is a fascinating one that deserves greater study.

for religious life. They belong together in the interests of better medical outcomes, as inclusion of a faith dimension fosters physical healing. They belong together in the interests of more fulfilling religious lives, since explicit integration of faith in the negotiation of physical trials enhances spiritual integrity and fulfilment.

When we say the two belong together, that belonging comes in three forms. Religion and medicine belong together *clinically*, to improve health outcomes and quality of life, informing the insights of doctors, patients, and spiritual leaders. When high-quality research indicates the effect of religious observance on all-cause mortality exceeds that of game-changing medications like statins such as atorvastatin, this is a connection that deserves attention on both medical and religious grounds.[2] If medicine needs spiritual sensitivity to activate the full range of healing resources, religion needs medical study to learn how best to apply its "broad spectrum" therapies, such as prayer and community. Faith needs this dialogue also to avoid the toxic side effects of some kinds of spirituality, which exist as surely as they do for pharmacological treatments.

The two belong together *descriptively* or analytically in the sense that when we look at major medical or religious developments, we often find hidden connections: religious dimensions to medical developments or medical aspects to religious ones. It is not possible to consider the history of the treatment of addiction without dealing with the Christian roots and spiritual dimension of twelve-step programs.[3] Even the rise of Christianity is a story entwined with the reality of plagues and healing.[4] Such looks backwards can alert us to aspects we may miss in our contemporary environment.

Third, religion and medicine belong together *reflectively*, as conversation partners. Thoughtful practitioners in either field find that their practice draws them into questions normally addressed in the other: a doctor drawn into consideration of the meaning of suffering and a pastor into consideration of the possible mechanisms of prayer's role in healing. Discussing medical topics (epidemics, cancer, pain, end of life) with voices from both communities draws out new perspectives and enriches each approach. It is the same with discussion of theological topics (incarnation, creation, resurrection, sin) when they are considered in a medical context. Medical

---

[2] See Chapter 6.
[3] See Chapter 9.
[4] See Chapter 7.

practitioners trying to assess health outcomes find themselves enmeshed in defining quality of life or assigning dollar amounts to a year of life, questions that are insoluble when isolated from orienting values that come from outside medicine itself. Religious adherents and leaders constantly find themselves immersed not in an abstract question of suffering, but in specific versions of it, some affected by genetics, some influenced by life choices, some traceable to environmental conditions. An assessment of the most faithful response to any particular condition often involves an appreciation of the best medical understanding of that condition.

For religious people to take medicine seriously means that medical information can affect religious evaluations. For medical people to take religion seriously means that spiritual resources are among the healing resources to be assessed and employed. Religious outlooks and medical ones must be in dialogue if each is to be authentic and relevant. Medicine without this dimension risks becoming a reductionist exercise. The body becomes a machine, illness a biological problem to be repaired. Life is measured in blood pressure, pulse, and respiratory rate. Religious reflection without engagement with medicine becomes too self-contained and abstract. We can ponder the nature of God's mind and variations in teaching among religious traditions, but lose touch with how faith helps us to heal, to live with suffering, and to approach the medical decisions around our own death.

We have found just this kind of mutual enrichment in our pastoral, clinical, and classroom experiences. This book aims to share some of that enrichment (and incite more) for patients reflecting on their own passage through the health care system and along the spiritual itinerary of their illness, for health care providers concerned to recognize the possibilities for enhanced healing, and for religious leaders who wish to support their people (including health care workers) in integrating faith and medicine. Though we seek to be honest about the real harm that can arise from tensions between spiritual commitments and medical perspectives or from forms of religion that are not good for health, our consistent theme is the promise for human healing we see in greater integration of the religious and medical dimensions.

Positive Shared Elements

All of us will need a physician at some point in life, some rarely and some often. All of us ask questions about life, love, and death, and need companions in that search. Some will associate directly with religious communities on that path, and many only at some remove. But the two, health and meaning, intertwine in every life.

What we might call "everyday" medicine and religion go about their businesses without any necessary apparent overlap, or any necessary conflict (which may be one of the reasons we tend to keep them mentally isolated). "Ordinary medicine" is vaccinations, broken bones set and mended, an antibiotic prescribed for an infection. The very routine successes of medicine mean that life flows on without great disruption or soul searching. "Ordinary religion," similarly, is worship, ritual, community, meaning-making, prayer for the sick: routine elements of someone's life whose cumulative effect (as we will see further on) may have major health implications, but which do not focus special attention on the medical world.

Medicine and religion meet more immediately at the extremes, both positive and negative. At the positive end, they meet in forms of wonder. A birth is an occasion of awe for the mother and family themselves, but a version of the same thing is felt by the obstetrician on a heightened level of understanding of the physiological detail and averted peril involved in any baby's arrival. That is not to mention the wonder felt by laypersons and professionals alike at instances of healing or recovery that defy medical expectation or accounting. There are joyous mysteries to be discovered in research on the extraordinary sophistication (and resilience) of our bodily natures that are not hard to connect with the Psalmist's awe at the depths of creation's complexity and order.

They meet also in negative extremes, where both encounter mysteries of ignorance and pain. For medicine, there is always the shadow of mortality, of fatal or chronic conditions that cannot be cured but only managed, of cases for which there is no clear cause and no clear treatment. All medical practitioners live to some extent in this zone of mystery and awe. For religious faith, there is always the shadow of evil and suffering, of questioning how these things relate to a divine source of hope and good. There is also the challenge of translating the conviction that religious practice intends to redeem this life, not only some future existence, into actual application to specific life experiences like illness.

How does healing happen? Anyone who has been at the bedside of a loved one has asked this question. Medicine pursues the question to its most intimate molecular and microscopic particulars. Spirituality seeks it even in the midst of and beyond the failure of all cures or treatments. The answer is always one of haunting humility and mystery. Even death can be a kind of healing. Cure is a medical term, as forgiveness or salvation are religious ones, but healing is a word that strikes the note they share, a holistic "making well."

In medicine, we can cut out a tumor, lower the blood pressure, and give antibiotics. In medicine, we treat the biological process of disease. Only recently, have medical schools incorporated more humanistic qualities into the curriculum: how to understand a patient's social determinants of health, how to break bad news to a family member. In theology, the diagnosis of brokenness and suffering becomes more complex: spiritual illness, alienation from the divine, fractured relationships with the community, nagging anxiety that the world is not right. In theology, physical illness is an important dimension of what ails us, but not the full or final story. As medicine has come to grapple with disease beyond the biologic model, so too has theology come to understand the importance of science in helping us sift and shape our spiritual traditions. Our bodies matter. And so do the beliefs, communities, and hopes that animate them.

The word "medicine" comes from the Latin verb to heal, *medeor*, with *medicina* referring to the substance given to the patient and *medicus* to the person doing the healing. The religious term salvation comes from the Latin *salvare*, to save, and its adjective *salvus*, well, unharmed, safe. There is the beautiful Hebrew concept of *tikkun olam*, which means "the healing of the world." As such language suggests, bodily well-being is decisively included in the religious vision, even used as an image for it. But that is an aspect of a more comprehensive reconciliation in which virtually all aspects of our world are subject to a hoped for change. Sickness, debility, suffering, and irrevocable death are not the world as it could or ought to be. Different religions have different diagnoses of how this state came to be and different regimes of belief and practice in how it may be overcome. The scope of such visions is vast, touching on things like social justice, economics, and psychology insofar as they figure in ultimate human flourishing.[5] The genius of medicine is its successful isolation of the special bio-physical aspect of that flourishing. But insofar as medicine follows the threads of our bodily

---

[5] Buddhism ascribes the root of human suffering to ignorant attachment to an impermanent phenomenal world. Muslims, Christians, and Jews describe an acquired "disease" of our nature, called sin, as the root of our broken relationships with God and each other. These religious traditions do not hesitate to describe their projects in "medical" terms, with prophets, bodhisattvas, or Christ cast as "great physicians" who treat what is comprehensively wrong with us.

illness out into the relationships, the social conditions, the environmental insults in which they are embedded, it moves toward dialogue with religion.

Medicine challenges theology to specify its relevance to physical healing. And theology breathes an expanded vision of well-being into medicine, going beyond simply ethical decision-making. The dialogue between the two grounds medicine in the philosophy and traditions of its rich humanistic heritage. The shared project of medicine and theology is the healing of the world.

Challenges

The estrangement of medicine and religion stems from forces in both areas. From the religious side, the most obvious form of conflict is belief in forms of divine healing as displacements for some or even all medical treatment. A religious person who sees much of medical science as an idolatrous competitor with direct divine action not only goes without the benefits of that science but reflects an oddly modern rupture with religion through the ages (and likely their own religious tradition), which was typically deeply integrated with what we would call medical techniques as well as ritual or spiritual ones.

Similarly, a medical provider who sees someone's religious ideation and commitments only as (at best) cultural oddities or (at worst) mental pathologies deserving treatment in their own right is unlikely to tap them as resources for healing. Based on real cases of religious resistance to medical treatment and real instances of mental illness expressed in religious idioms, providers can develop their own assumptions about religion as an intrinsic competitor with medicine, always an obstacle to be surmounted rather than a partner to be enlisted.

To some extent, the relations of religion and medicine stand in the shadow of wider cultural tensions between religion and science. Some, like Stephen Jay Gould, the celebrated Harvard biologist, advocated a "good fences make good neighbors" approach to that larger question. In his view, the two were "Non-Overlapping Magisteria": science answers questions about the internal functions of the universe and religion considers questions of meaning and transcendence.[6] Gould argued that each was best when it stayed in its lane

---

[6]Stephen Jay Gould, "Nonoverlapping Magisteria," *Natural History* 106 (1997): 16–22.

and did not interject itself into the other. The best relation was really no relation. We do not think this is a good prescription for science and religion in general, but it is out of the question for the concrete world of medicine, where science and faith meet in particular bodies and persons.

To say spirituality and medicine belong together does not imply that all medical providers or patients should be religious in any explicit way, that religion is a "treatment" to be applied to every ailment. Nor does it mean that religion's purpose and value are measured primarily by its health benefits. Rather, we would say spiritual outlook is a "vital sign," a key consideration. Like any vital sign—a temperature or a blood pressure reading—a spiritual reading will be more or less clinically relevant in a particular case. Just as you may be asked to rate your pain level on a ten point scale, or to respond to a questionnaire evaluating levels of depression or to an instrument assessing the extent of one's social supports, so too there is an important place for considering someone's operative convictions regarding meaning and ultimate reality. Such things may be indirectly involved in assessments of mental health or social support, but they deserve consideration in their own right.

There is such a thing as toxic religion, as there are iatrogenic (medical treatment-induced) illnesses. An old saying from pharmacology is "the dose makes the poison" and likewise the dose may make the cure. The right amount of potassium in your blood enhances health. An excess can stop your heart. Neither doctors or priests are used to thinking of religion in terms of "dosage." A major epidemiological study found attendance at religious services is associated with significant reduction in all cause mortality. It also indicated that this benefit attached to people who attend services at least once a month.[7] Higher attendance did not appear to add much mortality effect. "Take once a month" would be the directions if this were a prescription. But religious people are unlikely to modulate their behavior according to that kind of cost/benefit analysis, nor to regard the benefit in question as the ruling rationale for their behavior.

Just as there is no purely generic medicine, only specific diagnoses and specific treatments, so there is no brute amount of religion, a little or a lot. Rather, there are forms and aspects of religion. Traditional theological discourse has always focused not just on good or bad beliefs and practices,

---

[7] See Tyler VanderWeele et al., "Association of Religious Service Attendance with Mortality among Women." *Journal of the American Medical Association Internal Medicine* 176, no. 6 (2016): 777–85.

but also on distinguishing the right application of beliefs and practices. Serious consideration of religious influences on health outcomes will also have to address what kinds of religious practices and what aspects of religion are most relevant to particular outcomes.

Healthy Differences

Religious people are unlikely to calibrate their religious practice entirely for medical considerations, since there are other aims involved. And medicine cannot "prescribe" existential religious beliefs or committed practices that are not already consistent with a person's outlook. So another challenge for the medicine-theology conversation is to recognize this legitimate and healthy divergence. They are in fact distinct projects, and the tension between them is not always or simply the result of misunderstanding. Each is organized around aims that, while overlapping, cannot be subsumed one into the other. Medicine mainly seeks to heal bodies of their physical ailments, with all their personal entanglements. It is a corporeal, materialistic discipline informed by empirical evidence and partnered with (though not reducible to) science. Religion seeks to comprehensively heal persons, in their thoroughly bodily natures, in the wider context of their relationships, morals, and harmony with the divine.

For instance, the two diverge around their shared reference point of mortality. Medicine's entire concern is to fight the entropy of death, to establish health for the time being. Religion's concern extends to a wholeness (liberation, salvation, peace) transcending death or illness, and possibly even in the midst of them. Religious hope or commitment not only goes beyond health as medicine understands it, in the sense of adding something on top of it. That commitment may also relativize health itself, framing reasons that physical well-being or survival may not always be the ultimate priority. This is illustrated by a gerontologist who conducted an observational study of Hindu renunciants in India. They lived far below the poverty line. He found that their health ranged from "fair to quite poor," that they had no family support or friends. And yet he concluded "these men would have bumped the top of any scale of life satisfaction."[8]

---

[8] L. E. Thomas, "Dialogues with Three Religious Renunciates and Reflections on Wisdom and Maturity," *International Journal of Aging & Human Development* 32, no. 3 (1991): 225.

People may willingly put themselves at heightened risk to their health by virtue of religiously motivated service, practices, or travel. People may undertake ascetic activities that they regard as good for their spiritual lives even if not beneficial in a strict biological sense. Their commitment to serve their neighbors may put them at risk. Father Damien of Molokai is a famous example, a Catholic priest who went to work among the lepers of Hawai'i in their outcast villages and so himself eventually contracted and then died of the disease. In less dramatic ways, people often put fidelity to their understanding of the good life ahead of the optimal program in terms of stress, rest, diet, or access to medical care.

Two Languages for Healing

Another challenge in the conversation between medicine and religion is language. Medicine and theology use language differently. Medicine employs a very specific, exacting, narrow band language. Rather than the simple information that someone has a "rash," a doctor needs to know whether a patient has palpable purpura or maculopapular erythema. The first, "splotchy" and raised, may be a sign of an infection or a bleeding disorder and low platelets. The second, more differentiated, may be a more benign allergic reaction. The specific words matter because they lead to different diagnoses and treatments. What is more, the language is dense. If a fifty-five-year-old gentleman presents with difficulty breathing and has a history of congestive heart failure, chronic renal disease, and previously had cardiac stents placed followed by coronary bypass grafts in three vessels, a doctor would write, "55 yo male, presents with dyspnea, h/o CHF, CKD, CAD s/p PCI and CABGx3." This coded language is necessary to convey complex medical conditions, but it is completely impenetrable to the uninitiated. Every physician knows that for all their hard won knowledge, there is still a sea of ignorance about the body's functions and even about the mechanisms of action of standard therapies. But multivalent language of the mysterious and the ineffable, poetic language, has no useful place.

The language of religion is broad band, encompassing big ideas and poetic expression, subject to several levels of interpretation, and used in an enormous variety of contexts (ritual, song, teaching, worship). The language is performative or enactive in ritual: "I pronounce you husband and wife," "This is my body." It is direct address in prayer. It is prescriptive in moral or practical terms. It is poetic and evocative in song or litany. Religious people speak of sin, guilt, joy, grace, and forgiveness. These are (or have become) terms of everyday speech used widely by religious and non-religious people, overlapping with more specific religious explanations or definitions.

The premise of such language is that it refers, ultimately, to things that are not susceptible to exact description in our normal categories. Theistic religions recognize that a translation problem exists between human categories and divine realities. Indeed, the theological tradition invokes both a *cataphatic* way of approaching God—in which we build our understanding on descriptions of the divine according to our categories—and an *apophatic* way, which says we can come closer to the truth by emphasizing the way in which God is *not* grasped in our terms. In cataphatic terms it makes sense to think of God as "the great physician." But in apophatic terms, it also makes sense to think that divine healing or spiritual health cannot be equated with, might even negate, physical health. The unknown and mysterious are boundaries on the biological map that medical knowledge rightly seeks to push back, obstacles to better care. The incomprehensible excess in divine reality is a source of humility and hope in religious perception.

Religion does have its own dense and specialized language, drawn from thick narratives and from technical terms used by smaller numbers within traditions. In Christian theology, for instance, people discuss transubstantiation, transcendence, immanence, incarnation, and communion. Those in the early church argued whether Christ had one divine nature (*monophysitism*) or two natures, both divine and human (*dyophysitism*), and whether Christ was raised from the dead with a body. The early church pondered whether the Virgin Mary was the *Christokos* (Christ bearer) or the *Theotokos* (God bearer). Esoteric as such debates appear, there is no doubt that they were a medium for exploring human nature (including human biological nature) and the relation of spirit and body. If medicine emphasizes the exact, the specific, in its use of language, and religion encompasses both philosophical/metaphysical reflection and the simpler but layered language of scripture, ritual and devotion, how do we translate between the two? Wittgenstein, a philosopher of language, was vexed by such questions. In his *Philosophical Investigations*, he used the concept of God as an illustration.[9] When we use the word "God," one speaker

---

[9]See Ludwig Wittgenstein, *Philosophical Investigations: The English Text of the Third Edition* (New York: Macmillan, 1973). For a more explicit application of these ideas in theology, see George

may be invoking a benevolent creator akin to the metaphorical artistic figure in the Sistine Chapel, associated with wonder and awe. Another may use the word to refer to a malignant, capricious power who has inflicted unbearable suffering on their family member. The word "God" means vastly different things in the grammatically identical sentence used by two different people (or the same person at different times). Religious traditions are composed of tools, from texts to practices, to orient people in shared perspectives. This means that meaning is in significant part derived from use. The meaning of the word "God" is built up by following its employment through a set of scriptural texts, for example. Another avenue of orientation is by participation in shared acts of worship. The way someone deploys the idea of God tells us something about what it means. In this respect, we could say that exploring the use and effect of religious faith in medical contexts is one aspect of unpacking what religious terms mean.

Like the disciplines of medicine and theology themselves, their distinct languages tend to intersect at their depths. John Stone, a cardiologist-poet, addressed the graduating class of the medical school at Emory University in 1982. He tried to sum up for them the nature of the vocational life they had embarked upon. Titled *"Gaudeamus Igitur"* (Therefore Let Us Rejoice), Stone's address took its cue from medieval graduation ceremonies when university students would celebrate in the streets with singing. His poem captures well the themes of mystery and humility, suffering and joy, that he found in the life of the doctor. It reads in part:

> For this is the day you know too little
> > against the day when you will know too much
>
> For you will be invincible
> > and vulnerable in the same breath
> > which is the breath of your patients
>
> For their breath is our breathing and our reason
>
> For the patient will know the answer
> > you will ask him
> > ask her
>
> For the family may know the answer
>
> For there may be no answer
> > and you will know too little again

Lindbeck, *The Nature of Doctrine: Religion and Theology in a Postliberal Age* (Philadelphia: Westminster Press, 1984).

> or there will be an answer and you will know too much
> forever...
> For there is the mortar of faith
> For it helps to believe
> For Mozart can heal and no one knows where he is buried
> For penicillin can heal
> and the word
> and the knife
> For the placebo will work and you will think you know why
> For the placebo will have side effects and you will know
> you do not know why
> For none of these may heal
> For joy is nothing if not mysterious
> For your patients will test you for spleen
> and for the four humors
> For they will know the answer
> For they have the disease
> For disease will peer up over the hedge
> of health, with only its eyes showing
> For the T waves will be peaked and you will not know why...
>
> For the patient will live
> and you will try to understand
> For you will be amazed
> or the patient will not live
> and you will try to understand
> For you will be baffled
> For you will try to explain both, either, to the family
> For there will be laying on of hands
> and the letting go
> For love is what death would always intend if it had the choice.[10]

As Stone stretches to convey the nature of the vocation of medicine, the mystery of how healing happens (or does not), he is compelled to reach far beyond the language of medicine itself, to the humanistic world of poetry and religion. Even the technical language of medicine takes on additional levels of personal meaning. "T waves" are a feature seen in the visual tracing of an electrocardiogram. A particular "peaked" shape of the T wave is notoriously difficult to interpret. It could be associated with many different causes. For Stone, this term communicates to those with specialized familiarity not only

---

[10] John Stone, "Gaudeamus Igitur," *JAMA* 249, no. 13 (1983): 1741–2. Used by permission.

the literal meaning but a metaphorical one. For those who know the difficulties it poses, it is also a sign of mystery and the limits of medical knowledge.

Most striking, Stone's poem opens up the human narrative of the doctor. It does not tell the terse objective story of diagnosis and treatment, but the subjective inner itinerary of uncertainty, joy, frustration, and wonder that accompany the practice of medicine. It highlights the intense and asymmetrical connection between doctor and patient, where the patient "knows the answer" in the sense of having firsthand knowledge of their symptoms that the doctor must acquire from them, but the doctor knows the questions to which they are seeking the answers. Stone said of poetry, "it is one way of making sense of the world, and . . . it has the power to heal."[11]

In the age of Shakespeare, Anglican priest John Donne offered a kind of mirror image to Stone's reflection as a medical practitioner. In his poem *Hymn to God, My God, in My Sickness*, Donne spoke from the perspective of a patient, from the bed of what was perhaps his terminal illness.

> Since I am coming to that Holy room,
>   Where, with Thy choir of saints for evermore,
> I shall be made Thy music; as I come
>   I tune the instrument here at the door,
>   And what I must do then, think here before;
>
> Whilst my physicians by their love are grown
>   Cosmographers, and I their map, who lie
> Flat on this bed, that by them may be shown
>   That this is my south-west discovery,
>   *Per fretum febris*,[12] by these straits to die;
>
> I joy, that in these straits I see my west;
>   For, though those currents yield return to none,
> What shall my west hurt me? As west and east
>   In all flat maps—and I am one—are one,
>   So death doth touch the resurrection . . .
>
> We think that Paradise and Calvary,
>   Christ's cross and Adam's tree, stood in one place;

---

[11]Quoted in Anne Hudson Jones, "Literature and Medicine: Physician-Poets," *The Lancet* 349, no. 9047 (1997): 278.
[12]Latin "by the strait of fever."

> Look, Lord, and find both Adams met in me;
>   As the first Adam's sweat surrounds my face,
>   May the last Adam's blood my soul embrace.[13]

From Donne we hear a patient's narrative: not the medical analysis of his disease or even a first-person account of his symptomatic experience, but the story of what his illness *means* to him.[14] To Donne's attentive physicians, with their "geographical" knowledge, the body is a map, and healing is an act of navigation. Those currents of illness "yield return to none." The physicians' map is organized by the medical framework of their times. But patients overlay this with a map that expresses their subjective experience. When someone speaks of their cancer as an "invader" or of "fighting off" an infection, they reflect the way that they are imagining and understanding what is happening. Donne frames his illness in the wider mysteries, of death and resurrection, of how the faith in Christ that has guided his whole life will carry him through its final "straits." His sick room is a "Holy room," for the medical treatment finally gives way to another kind of healing: reconciliation and hope.

Historians are unsure whether the poem was written during an illness (perhaps typhus fever) from which Donne recovered, or in fact during his final sickness. That ambiguity reflects the fact that the religious dimension is often integral to the holistic care that medicine increasingly understands plays a role in physical healing, but that it is always a part of a patient's response to the limitations of physical healing and the search for ultimate peace.

As these two examples show, theology and medicine meet in persons. They meet within the person of the healer and within the person of the patient, as well as within the relationship between them. For it is in these places that both sickness and health take on their lived meaning. And those meanings are often themselves a medium for healing.

---

[13] John Donne, *John Donne: The Complete English Poems* (London: Penguin Classic 1977). 347.
[14] The importance of the patient's perspective on illness is regularly rediscovered. See Susan Sontag, *Illness as Metaphor*, 1st Vintage Books ed. (New York: Vintage Books, 1979); Norman Cousins, *Anatomy of an Illness as Perceived by the Patient: Reflections on Healing and Regeneration* (New York: Norton, 1979). Often it is artists and writers who give accounts of their own experiences. But in an even wider sense novelists regularly turn to disease as a central metaphor for wider accounts of the human condition, as in Albert Camus, *The Plague* (Geneva,: Edito-Service S.A., 1974).

References

Camus, Albert. *The Plague.* Geneva: Edito-Service S.A., 1974.

Cousins, Norman. *Anatomy of an Illness as Perceived by the Patient: Reflections on Healing and Regeneration.* New York: Norton, 1979.

Donne, John. *John Donne: The Complete English Poems.* London: Penguin Classic, 1977.

Gould, Stephen Jay. "Nonoverlapping Magisteria." *Natural History* 106 (1997): 16–22.

Jones, Anne Hudson. "Literature and Medicine: Physician-Poets." *The Lancet* 349, no. 9047 (1997): 275–8.

Lindbeck, George. *The Nature of Doctrine: Religion and Theology in a Postliberal Age.* Philadelphia: Westminster Press, 1984.

Sontag, Susan. *Illness as Metaphor.* 1st Vintage Books ed. New York: Vintage Books, 1979.

Stone, John. "Gaudeamus Igitur." *JAMA* 249, no. 13 (1983): 1741–2.

Thomas, L. E. "Dialogues with Three Religious Renunciates and Reflections on Wisdom and Maturity." [In English]. *International Journal of Aging & Human Development* 32, no. 3 (1991): 211–27.

VanderWeele, Tyler, Li Sharshan, Meir J. Stampfar, and David R. Williams. "Association of Religious Service Attendance with Mortality among Women." *Journal of the American Medical Association Internal Medicine* 176, no. 6 (2016): 777–85.

Wittgenstein, Ludwig. *Philosophical Investigations; the English Text of the Third Edition.* New York: Macmillan, 1973.

2

The Wound of Mortality
Theology and Medicine in the Anatomy Lab

Chapter Outline	
The Wound of Mortality	19
Calling and Obligation	26
The Face of the Calling	30

Twenty-seven metal tables range in two rows down a long open space, like three large classrooms end to end. At each table, gowned and gloved first-year nursing students busily retract stainless steel covers, revealing heavy plastic bags whose zippers open to expose one waxy, yellowish-grey, human body. On the wall, posted like a caption in a museum, an index to the numbered tables gives a few basic facts about this person: age, cause of death, major medical conditions.

Three or four nurses in training gaze at a computer screen extended on a long arm to hover above their body, trying to match what they see there with the cadaver below. They click through amazingly vivid virtual images of the contents of the throat and upper chest in a ruddy healthy textbook body, while searching with their fingers in the chemical-scented, rubbery flesh.

Scattered beside them at their islands today are a class of seminary students. For a few of them—health professionals in a prior career—this marks a return to a familiar setting. For most, it is like entering a secret kingdom where a child's curiosity may peer and poke behind the curtain of our flesh. Most hidden veins of life are uncovered to us sooner rather than later. We learn the depths of grief by sad experience. We are initiated into intimate or forbidden physical acts by pornographies of sex and violence. But the realm of the dead stays shadowed still, preserved in relative privacy by some combination of professional boundaries, lingering reverence, and lack of urgent entertainment value. As modern medical patients, we are awash in the spectral pictures of our inner life, from X-rays and ultrasounds to CAT scans and MRIs. Those black-and-white digital images are ghosts, not bodies. What lies before us is quite different.

Some divinity students lean forward into the circle, eager to be invited to touch and feel within the neat wounds opened by the dissector's knife. Others stand uncertainly to the side. One student holds another's hand as they edge nearer to the table. The bodies are in different stages of disassembly. Some have become heaps of piled pieces—lungs, heart, liver—detached and examined separately. As living bodies wear out and wear down, so do these remnant ones. They bear scattered vestiges of past interventions: pacemakers, hip implants, knee replacements, bypass grafts. Before the class is ended, the cases zipped and closed for the night, all the parts will be reassembled and resettled, an instinctive gesture at repair and a courtesy to the next explorers.

The conversations flow readily, as our groups are somewhat mirror images of each other. Resident students focus on learning what they most need to learn, and for them, a whole range of questions slide into their private thoughts or off times. They press aside nagging concerns—are our hearts thickening like this one, our lungs hardening like that?—with a professional one: how to find that particular artery or physiological junction in some future urgent medical need.

For us it is the reverse. We have no practical need for this knowledge, only existential questions. What does it matter to know that this is me: I have one of those, two of these, and am only separated in time from being this heap of parts? What does it mean to hold a heart or a brain in your hand and think at the same time of creation, God, resurrection? Our perspectives crisscross each other. A divinity student asks the anatomy teaching assistant, "Can you tell whether this person lived a good life?" wondering whether diet, exercise, and adherence to medical wisdom can be read off the cadaver like a final exam. The somewhat puzzled assistant replies, "Isn't that something that's more in your department to decide?"

The Wound of Mortality

Mortality is a universal wound at the heart of medicine and religion. It is an overarching shadow on human life, pervasive if sometimes dim, conditioning all our visions of meaning and good. It bleeds tangibly when we face the eruption of specific injuries or diseases and their attendant anxieties, occasions when the wound is concretely evident and reluctantly acknowledged with others. In every emergency room and doctor's office, the vast majority of daily events repeat a sacrament of assuaged fear. The rash, the headache, the fever, are judged to be harmless or reparable. The intimation that these might portend something more ominous, even the very end itself, recedes. But this is a holding action, and all parties know it. The liturgy of the medical life is full of celebration: the well baby visit, the happy test result, the yearly check up with good advice for years to come. The life of ministry has its baptisms and weddings, spiritual growth, transforming service, and festal worship. But the line from the Book of Common Prayer's burial service stands in equal, measure over both: "In the midst of life we are in death."

The anatomy lab is both the beginning and the end of the medical journey, the start of the study and the brute fact of its limit. Nothing could seem to teach the dichotomy of spirit and body more than this. The cadavers are aggressively inert and material. The bodies that hover over them, alight with energy and purpose, are not. But even here, the temple of the "mere" body, the two are always blending into each other. The body at the center of medicine, even when isolated and de-personed, yet remains an experienced body. In this case it is experienced by us, and that experience includes the projected presence of the one whose body it is or has been. At every turn in the path of illness, it is often hard to tell whether the most profound suffering is located more in the one (the biological body) or the other (the experiential body). So, too, with the healing.

The intimate dance of obligation and vulnerability that shadows the medical world is already underway in this space, even without living patients. Here on the tables, one source of religion itself lies bare at the root. That root is a mute question posed by the bodies of our own kind, a question that has aroused millennia of response. It is in those earliest burials, where we can discern the signs of other-care for injuries and hopeful concern for the departed, that we register the flickers of a humanity like our own.

Indeed, it is reverence for the body as inseparable from the spirit that long stood in the way of what happens here. In the Western world until the fifteenth century, the dissection of human beings was popularly considered a desecration. Even though church authorities in many places allowed it for the purpose of study, it was rare. But by the time of Vesalius' masterwork *De humani corpora's Fabrica Libra septem* (1543), it was becoming a widespread element in medical education.[1] This led to a scramble to procure sufficient bodies for the practice. For centuries these derived predominantly from executed criminals (for whom dissection was an additional punishment) and the poor (whether by appropriation or direct purchase).[2]

Even the presence of these bodies in the lab has a religious history. The population in the anatomy lab is not religiously random. Missing are those whose traditions call for immediate burial, or for ritual treatments that make the cadavers unsuitable, or which forbid mutilation of the body. The appreciation of the educational value of dissection had to go hand in hand with religious understandings. Popular ideas of the resurrection of the dead (and a desire to preserve bodies intact pursuant to that hope) militated against dissection, even though theological teachings did not in principle distinguish dissection from the many other forms of disintegration to which bodies were subject. The objection was often less to the damage to the resurrection hopes of the dead than to the disrespect dissection might suggest to the deceased person and the divine handiwork of the body.[3] The biblical view that the good creation was a material one, that bodies testified to divine order and were destined themselves for a kind of redemption could be taken both as a charter of reverence toward the body and as an invitation to investigate the manner in which humans are "fearfully and wonderfully made."[4]

Some in the medical field suggest such labs have outlived their usefulness and everything they teach can be better learned by computers and simulation. Its defenders point to the technical benefits of idiosyncratic realism: there

---

[1] The Library of Congress provides an online version of a 1555 edition. Andreas Vesalius, *On the Fabric of the Human Body in Seven Books* (Basel, Switzerland: Joannes Oporinus, 1555). https://hdl.loc.gov/loc.wdl/wdl.19493.

[2] SK Ghosh, "Human Cadaveric Dissection: A Historical Account from Ancient Greece to the Modern Era," *Anatomy & Cell Biology* 48, no. 3 (2015). 157–61.

[3] Over time, the "reassembly" image of resurrection found in some parts of scripture tended to give way to another, Pauline image of the risen spiritual body as something new grown from the "seed" of the deceased body. See Caroline Walker Bynum, *The Resurrection of the Body in Western Christianity, 200–1336*, Lectures on the History of Religions; New Ser., No. 15 (New York: Columbia University Press, 1995).

[4] Psalm 139:14. I praise you, for I am fearfully and wonderfully made. Wonderful are your works; that I know very well. NRSV updated version.

are no generic hearts, only actual ones. But they clearly intimate something less tangible, something students gain from beginning with a paradoxical relationship where, as one student put it, "We . . . are training to make people whole again, yet we treat our first patient by taking them fully and irrevocably apart."[5] This is a spiritual lab too, where medical students begin to seek their peace with the failure that finally attends their efforts and the fears that their failures could hasten, not postpone, that end.

A body bare, dead, and undefended, calls forth in us a well of responses that are not clinical: reflexive embarrassment on behalf of those so rudely open to our gaze and touch, fear and anxiety over our own mortality, triggered pain from losses past, sober tremors over the depth of what is at stake. The donors here are without exception elderly people, and our fantasies of them can revolve around that encouraging fact, at least. One student asks whether the bodies of any young adults or children are ever used for this basic instruction. The answer is simple. "No, that would be too hard." It is not a medical judgment, but a human one.

The first day in class, the instructors tell us, nothing is done on the medical front. It is time for adjustment, to cope with the human emotions they must learn to set aside to do their professional work. One professor gives everyone paper and pen and asks them to draw a body or some aspect of it. So doctors and nurses begin their practice of filtering normal human responses and self-referential rumination in favor of the interpretive attentiveness that serves their calling. The minister or spiritual counselor likewise needs to cultivate a focused presence, a distance that serves empathy and care, but preserves emotional balance and insight.

There is something about this experience that seems to spontaneously call forth an almost liturgical response, an expression of gratitude and awe. Different medical schools have different traditions to honor the human as well as technical dimensions of relation with the donors. An important aspect of the Yale anatomy lab is found in the hallway outside the dissection room. The hallway is adorned with deeply moving paintings, drawings, poems, testimonials, and other works of art produced by students with reference to the persons whose bodies they have studied. This threshold display signals that one is entering a sacred space. The students know the important gift these people have made of themselves in their dying.

---

[5]Kathryn E. Norman, "This Is My Body," *Journal of the American Medical Association* 320, no. 5 (2018): 441.

At the end of the year, there is a service of recognition, and those that "belong" to one of the bodies write letters of appreciation to their unnamed donor. Some of these end up posted in the hallway. Elsewhere, medical schools have arranged for the students to receive letters written by the donors before their deaths. Many of those express the motivation behind the decision: a teacher saying in this way she will continue to teach after she dies, a donor to a Taiwan medical school writing "may you make a thousand mistaken cuts on my body, to avoid even one mistaken one on the living."

The road to healing begins with a donation, a gift from a nameless patient. This is a kind of afterlife. Not a resurrection, but a tangible lingering of the body to mutely testify and teach. For this season, they are the teachers, to whom the care giver stands in debt. The body of the patient is the door to practical knowledge. But it also teaches wonder. The opened body "holds an order and a beauty that I could not have imagined, one that I now realize is also within me and my laboratory partners and the people I love and the people I don't."[6]

A senior professor traces for us the arterial system through which this female body had nourished the child it bore long ago. She points out the still distinguishable point in this person's heart where, upon her own birth, and the first breath of air into newborn lungs, the hole that had allowed the mother's oxygenated blood to pass freely between the right and left ventricle now closed. Awe is still audible in her explanation of the sequence through which the two systems function and then dramatically disengage, like a lunar module and its mother ship.

The body teaches thankfulness, recalling to one student the words she had long heard around another table, where gift and gratitude impel a response of service. "I hold her heart in my hand, arteries and veins neatly severed, windows cut so that I can see the valves inside. 'This is my body broken for you. Do this in remembrance of me.'"[7]

Two Professions

These two ancient professions, healer and priest, long intertwined in a shamanistic middle field where physical restoration and immersion in the

---

[6]Ibid.
[7]Ibid.

spirit world cohere. "Religion and medicine have been in alliance with each other in every land, among all peoples, and almost throughout the entire course of recorded human history."[8] Ultimate well-being and order intersected seamlessly with the fate of our physical selves. Attempt to isolate spirit and body as we may in some of our philosophies and spiritualities, the integration persists. No spiritual leader lacks for requests to aid with physical healing, and no medical professional escapes inquiries as to meaning and the transcendent.

Spirits and bodies touch more obviously at their extremities. Their articulation in our daily lives is likely to go as unremarked as that between the components of our joints, absent some pain or dysfunction. A healthy mind in a healthy body may be a recipe for happy forgetfulness of the links between them, leaving us free to be absorbed by the projects of the whole person in the world, by the exaltations in which the sensory and the spiritual are always mixed. There are religious experiences born of overflowing joy and gratitude, religious outlooks driven not to fix what is broken but to find glory in the mundane. In medicine, it is a relatively recent development that seeks not only rescue from illness and disease but facilitation of peak performance and well-being. Sports medicine, cosmetic surgery, medication to enhance our cognitive capacities: these all push health care explicitly in the direction where healing gives way to flourishing, to serving the realization of what we understand to be the good or the best life. Nevertheless, we tend to attend more to our bodies and spirits as broken than as perfected. The path of the "twice born," whose spiritual journey runs through a valley of loss and brokenness, is relevant for us all. Illness, chronic or intermittent, marks the constant fact that we are debtors to death. This truth and its awareness are prompts for all religion, as they are the inescapable horizon of medicine's long, losing war against entropy.

Medicine is committed to winning as many battles as possible in the losing cause, and religion seeks to come to terms with the final calculus in a way that informs daily life. People in perfect health whose life is barren of purpose, joy, or hope are not well. The medical treatment offered in such cases, in the line of mental health, verges necessarily toward the religious. People in debilitating illness, however firm their spiritual perspective, seek

---

[8] Rabbi Immanuel Jakobovits, quoted in Jeffrey S. Levin, *Religion and Medicine: A History of the Encounter between Humanity's Two Greatest Institutions* (New York: Oxford University Press, 2020). Xvi.

and hope for concrete care and cure. The language of health, like that of justice or peace is often used in religious traditions to describe a final state, pointing to something for which the healing and resumption of our mortal lives can only be a kind of promissory taste. In a narrow medical view it is that contingent restoration of bodily health that is the defining aim, and religious or spiritual attitudes or practices are understandably viewed in light of their contribution to that end.

If sickness often marks the awareness of the wound of mortality in our daily lives, one part of religion is an attempt to weave our lives themselves around a response to, a "treatment" of that wound. Medicine strives to overcome finitude in a temporal frame: healing at the retail level, we might say. Faith seeks to overcome it in a more existential one. It not only directly faces the final fact, but it addresses the distinct problem of what it means to live successfully during both our long term as well as short term dying. It is healing at the wholesale level, we might say.[9] When we are faced with deadly illness and a certain term to our lives, the pressure intensifies to say what is meaningful to us, by what guide we will order the decisions remaining to us. As people in such circumstances regularly remind us, there is nothing special about this condition or its questions except temporal focus. It is our universal and constant state.

In the catalog of intense religious experiences, where we find those of unrestricted and overwhelming gratitude, or of unitary, boundary-less joy, one characteristic entry is the piercing perception of our mortality. Unsoftened by distraction, the certainty and clarity of our finitude comes home with such power that "normal" life seems hollow. It is not uncommon for religious traditions to describe themselves, in part, as preparation for death. The young prince who would become the Buddha had such a moment of clarity and challenge, encountering a corpse beside the road. Because he could not unsee what the corpse meant, he set out to seek a way to end all suffering. Jesus' followers, huddled in perplexity and despair after his execution, encountered him in life beyond death. In this light, they reordered their world. Sickness, pain, incapacitation, and death are often prompts for reorientation. In these particular cases, the reorientations became world-wide movements.

---

[9] See Miroslav Volf, Matthew Croasmun, and Ryan McAnnally-Linz, *Life Worth Living: A Guide to What Matters Most* (New York: The Open Field/Penguin Life, 2023).

The spheres of suffering are also liminal spaces from which we might emerge transformed and changed. No small number of students in our classes arrive impelled by just such experiences. These may be experiences (on the part of the student or someone close to them) of miraculous or spiritually enhanced healing. Just as often, they are experiences of chronic, intractable suffering. Indeed, we have had students whose weekly attendance at or absence from class tracked their hospitalizations and incapacitations with wrenching disease.

Just as students come from either end of a personal health spectrum, they come equally from those on the "medical" and the "religious" academic tracks. This mirrors the experience that each of us had individually prior to our collaboration. That is, Ben has seen a steady trickle of former ministers or ministerial students pursuing healthcare careers, saying they felt limited in their pastoral path and turned to medicine in the hope of concretely helping people. They remarked on an admiration approaching envy for the capacity of doctors and nurses to set a bone, relieve pain, or cure an illness, while their spiritual work was so often hard to quantify or confirm.

Mark likewise has seen a steady trickle in the reverse direction. These were nurses and physicians coming to divinity school, who spoke with frustration at the limits of their capacity to really help people, of the people whose chronic conditions they could not overcome or those for whom they could write a prescription or perform a successful surgery, but who left the office or hospital for a life where the same or worse would quickly happen again, for reasons they were powerless to affect: loneliness, financial destitution, loss of family or human connection, despair and hopelessness. Despite the profound accomplishments of medical knowledge, oftentimes the path to health is blocked by factors far outside its control.

A former seminary colleague noted that from the medical side of the aisle, the unique advantage of the treatment modalities of religion was glaringly obvious.[10] Those modalities include community and spiritual nourishment, two things desperately needed for healing, but beyond the capacity of medicine to provide. The colleague worked tirelessly to awaken pastors and congregations to the full scope of the superpower that was proper to their nature, rather than pining after the technology of medicine. What congregations do daily is pray constantly for the sick, both people

---

[10] B.L. Gill-Austern, "Rediscovering Hidden Treasures for Pastoral Care," *Pastoral Psychology* 43 (1995): 233–53.

known by particular name and face, as well as "all the sick" in all conditions. In addition, congregations do everything the doctor would prescribe if only they could but cannot: transportation to and from the appointment, meals when the patient is home, help with finances, attention to whether someone is doing what is advised, in terms of diet, or simply getting medicine the last three feet from container to mouth. This is not to mention the crucial activity of walking with a person in all the human processing of their condition, its emotional, and familial, and spiritual meaning for them and those they love.

There is no substitute for the wisdom shared in a twenty-minute doctor's appointment every few weeks or the life-changing skill exercised in surgical procedures. And there is no substitute for the supports of community and inner meaning that can sustain an individual through the twenty-four hour and seven-day-a-week world of anxiety, uncertainty, and pain that fills the time between medical interventions. We are acutely aware that just as there is an ideal of optimal medical care combined with healing spiritual support, reality can often demonstrate either dysfunctional medical care or counterproductive religious influences, and even both. These point us to different sides of what truly helping means, and each stands out more powerfully from the perspective of the other. These two sides of the coin are very deeply connected, but too rarely and haphazardly so in explicit practice. There are many attempts to put back together what cannot effectively be so radically divided. [11]

Calling and Obligation

Ministry and medicine are vocations marked by special ethics. Indeed, our cultural concept of a "profession," melding as it does mastery of some set of specialized skills with thorough devotion to a higher, selfless purpose, is essentially modeled on these two cases.[12] Those attracted to the medical professions may tend toward a psychological "problem solver" profile and those attracted to the pastoral professions may tend toward a psychological "nurturing" profile. But there are many kinds of problem solvers and helpers,

---

[11] See for instance Chapter 4 "Congregations and Communities," in Levin, *Religion and Medicine: A History of the Encounter between Humanity's Two Greatest Institutions*.

[12] See Charles R. Foster, *Educating Clergy: Teaching Practices and the Pastoral Imagination*, 1st ed. (San Francisco: Jossey-Bass, 2006). 194–5.

ranging from engineers to child care givers. It is not just personality and task definition that define these paths. They function within the scope of a peculiar kind of obligation, a responsibility that they purposely assume and which is also projected on them by those they serve.

In this sense, medicine and ministry are not "jobs." In both instances, those vested with special gifts or skills become stewards who, in turn, have a commensurate obligation. The administration of those gifts does not belong to their personal determination alone. It is a function of a "calling." For religious leaders, the calling and obligation come explicitly from beyond themselves: from God and the religious community. And insofar as the earliest healers attributed the value in their treatments to divine actions or a legacy of transmitted wisdom, they fit the same pattern. Coordinate with the idea that such activities were not just a way to make a living or the property of individuals who invented or acquired them, was the expectation that they should be administered in an other-directed as opposed to a selfish manner.

Long before physicians had much in the way of surgical and pharmacological resources that might dramatically alter the course of their patients' health, their discipline was distinguished as much by its ethos as by its technique.[13] What set them apart was an existential, unrestricted commitment to put the well-being of the patient ahead of any personal interest or the service of other masters. In addition to knowledge, what the physician offered was human qualities, including a purity of attention and loyalty, a promise to guard privacy, to resist conflict of interest, and to defer to the freedom of the patient to define outcomes, including what counts as healing. This meant not to use their knowledge to do ill to one on behalf of another (poisoning, for instance) or to do positive harm to the health of their patient, even at their invitation. Within the scope of those obligations, the doctor was to honor the choices of their patients, to accept their ordering of goods rather than imposing their own. In this respect, "bedside manner" was close to the totality of medical practice and care was an inescapably personal, face to face reality. In today's somewhat disjointed practice of medicine, it is often hard to know where to expect these qualities to be exercised. And yet they remain central to the vocational self-understanding of doctors and the expectations of their patients.

---

[13]See William F. May, *The Physician's Covenant: Images of the Healer in Medical Ethics*, 2nd ed. (Lexington, KY: Westminster John Knox Press, 2000).

Priests and ministers have been set apart, and for similarly differentiated reasons. They were also thought to be required to put their own interests second to those they served, to maintain confidences, and to avoid harm. But the requirement stemmed first from their obedience to divine power and second from their authorization/recognition on behalf of the community. Their "skill" was intimate knowledge of the divine resources, custodianship of the rituals and teachings that could benefit others. Their obligation was to the ultimate well-being of those they served, a well-being that could and ultimately did diverge from physical health. They could "prescribe" paths of behavior whose outcome was decreased health and even death, as preferable to behaviors deemed destructive to one's spirit, soul, or religious integrity. They majored in concern for hope and meaning precisely where these are most threatened in the shadows of bodily failing and death.

The two vocations are now distinct. Yet there is partial convergence in the sense that both stand under an imperative that comes from beyond themselves. That imperative comes mediated through the presence of the neighbor, and most especially the needy neighbor. The foundation for specialized medical and spiritual "workers" lies in something that is not special to these professions, an imperative toward a universal human mutuality. What Christians and Jews view as the two great commandments—to love God and love your neighbor—summarize that obligation. The trained doctor, the communally empowered religious leader, begin with the call that rests on every person or every member of a religious community: the basic care of their neighbor.

What a person owes their neighbor, or what love of God impels for their neighbor, is immediate, non-technical. We see it manifest in our instinctive flinch at an impending injury to another or the spontaneous impulse to well-wishing or prayer for those suffering or distraught. The almost reflexive version of this care—the hand extended instinctually to one who stumbles, the rush to seize a child from danger—falters as the needs and their responses become more extended and complex. The universal imperative fades before our differential care for those closest to us, and in face of ills that extend in structure and time beyond the scope of immediate personal response. Yet one distinctive feature of medicine and ministry is the respect in which their self-understandings depend upon concrete formulation of that universal impulse.

The quality of this obligation to our neighbor is universal, but its specific content can differ by capacity. While almost everyone may have a spontaneous hand to offer to a falling person, only some have specialized knowledge or office. For them, there is a new dimension to this simple, normal love of neighbor. As you would not deny a hand, would you not deny your specialized aid, which is only, as it were, a longer arm or a stouter pole with which to assist the drowning person? To obtain medical or spiritual capacities is to incur a greater liability, in this respect. We express this sensibility when someone falls ill on a plane or in a theatre and those in authority ask "Is there a doctor in the house?" This expresses not only a need, but an expectation. For one to acknowledge the identity is to acknowledge a responsibility. A parallel impulse arises at the time of death (or in the presence of what is clearly extreme spiritual anguish), when people look around the circle seeking someone ready to stand forward with ritual, prayer or counsel. Any of us would, and should, do as best we might in such situations. But training and preparation singles some out to bear the obligation foremost.

To say that health care is a "human right" takes us down troubled paths of political and social thought. But such an idea is both theoretically and historically inseparable from the sense of obligation we have been discussing: what is available to the physician is owed to those who need it, as what is entrusted to the minister is owed to those it can help. The right does not inhere in the one who suffers, but in the one whose obligation is not to turn away. Better, we could say, it rests on the reality of healing as interhuman encounter, which generates its own intrinsic responsibilities and evokes the divine commandment of love of neighbor.

The flip side of this obligation is found in the tacit human claim posed by the vulnerability of the neighbor in need. Such vulnerability can be helpless and unwilling: we fall unable to cure or care for ourselves. But it always includes a possible further voluntary dimension. What is granted to physician and priest—access to our bodies and knowledge of our private conditions and behaviors in the first case, access to our inner lives as well as knowledge of our private behaviors in the other—can impel a sense of responsibility in return. It is under the hope of this trust, belief in such a prior obligation, that the patient may be willing to "bare all," in the concrete sense of allowing intimate access to their body, or to the equally intimate confession of their true experiences and actions. We look to our doctors to glean from us information we are not aware is important to our well-being (is the pain sharper on our intake of breath than on the outflow?), but we possess relevant knowledge we may not readily divulge unless confident in nonmedical trust and understanding (we have done things we are not proud of and do not want others to know).

Strict confidentiality, an unrestricted commitment to put the patient above the expectations of employers, and even above one's own selfish interest—these are not "treatment" in the narrow sense, but are essential in what distinguishes doctors from technicians or contractors. Beneath all the paperwork, the interposition of insurance companies and government agencies, the relation of doctor and patient still bears the imprint of an elemental, primordial encounter, between a mute, fragile, suffering body on one side and on the other a fellow person who, by dint of special wisdom or special calling cannot turn away. That ethos, and the patient's trust in it, is part of what makes healing possible. [14]

The Face of the Calling

In some anatomy labs, a thin cloth lies across the faces of the donors. It preserves, for all but those times of actual study, a vestige of the reserve of clothing. A reticence intuitively extends to the face even more than to the genitals. Perhaps the gesture means to spare us the slightly uncanny sense that the donors are looking back at us, or the embarrassment we imagine on their behalf at being observed unaware or helpless. It reflects a respect for their individuality and personhood, which we associate above all with these unique physical windows of our humanity. This quirk of the anatomy lab has resonance with the responsibility intrinsic to these two callings.

It is no accident that philosophers and theologians, thinking far from this explicit medical space, should fix on the body as a site of ultimacy, as speaking to us in an elemental way. And in the body, it is above all the face that is given this speaking quality. Scripture says that to "know as we are known" is paradigmatically to "see face to face."[15] Faces, through which we read each other's thoughts and emotions most powerfully, communicate an implicit claim for attention and response. They can be theatres of conflict and

---

[14] The "Hippocratic" oath is one historical expression of this dimension of medicine. One may argue that this highly idealistic view of the practice puts impossible demands upon the physician and plays no small role in physician burnout. See F. Jotterand, "The Hippocratic Oath and Contemporary Medicine: Dialectic between Past Ideals and Present Reality?" *Journal of Medical Philosophy* 30, no. 1 (2005): 107–28. However, many physicians feel that some version of this self-understanding is what drew them to medicine and is the source of much of the satisfaction they take in its practice.
[15] 1 Corinthians 13:12.

rejection, but they are the archetypical media of comfort, reconciliation, encouragement and acceptance: windows of healing encounter.

Emmanuel Levinas famously reflected on the human face as an index to our most fundamental human obligations. Our morality, he suggested, cannot be abstracted into a rational calculus of abstract obligations, separated from its relational context. Our capacity for moral reflection always includes the imaginative vision of our own behavior or thoughts laid open to the sight and knowledge of others. We can rationalize behaviors which we are yet ashamed to picture performing before our neighbors' faces. For Levinas, seeing and being seen mediates the basic phenomena of embarrassment and shame, of involuntary revulsion and spontaneous care, in which we cringe from the sight of hurtful impact on another body or reflexively move to shield a child.

That is to say, we rightly experience the presence of another person's face as the expression of a command or obligation. The presence of the neighbor can be seen as the mediation, the activation, of the divine command to love that flows to us from above. Or that presence can evoke a mutuality of human connection whose imperative draws us beyond the mundane.

For Levinas, the presence of the other, embodied in their face, implies an implicit obligation, whose unconditioned character has a divine quality.

> The first word of the face is the "Thou shalt not kill." It is an order. There is a commandment in the appearance of the face, as if a master spoke to me. However, at the same time, the face of the Other is destitute; it is the poor for whom I can do all and to whom I owe all. [16]

This felt obligation comes to us partly through our awareness of each other as mortal. The faces and bodies we present to each other are mute testimony to that shared reality. The anatomy lab affects us on this frequency, tuned to a rare intensity. There we see both the uniqueness of each of us in bare, bodily form, and the simultaneous solidarity of us all in the same inert dependence. These things are conveyed by the bodies themselves. The emotional valence of being together in the presence of these others has a tint of nostalgia, as if we all had the same hometown or spoke the same mother tongue. We sense our unity with those on the tables, and, tenderly, with each other, like a wry, furtively exchanged smile: "You too."

---

[16] Emmanuel Lévinas and Philippe Nemo, *Ethics and Infinity*, 1st ed. (Pittsburgh: Duquesne University Press, 1985), 89.

Of course, Levinas writes,

> We have the power to relate ourselves to the other as an object, to oppress and exploit him; nevertheless the relation to the other, as a relation of responsibility, cannot be totally suppressed ... Here it is impossible to free myself by saying "It is not my concern." There is no choice, for it is always and inescapably my concern.[17]

The human face is simply the clearest window on this condition, a sight whose meaning we implicitly grasp as a question we must answer. Our encounter with each other's faces, Levinas suggests, itself communicates something on the same metaphysical level as divinity. He does not define God as a supreme being but as the supreme other, a supreme "being-for-the-other." Relation with such a God is necessarily a three way operation, for "is divinity possible without relation to a human other?"[18]

Medicine and religion work in the explicit theater of death. Each concrete area of intersection or divergence between them is mapped within this horizon. And each calling responds to a face-to-face imperative that is manifest to us in the bodily weakness of our neighbors. This is the nature of the obligation conveyed by the bodies in the anatomy lab when they lived, and which they express still. They reveal the open wound of mortality and claim its healing as a common task, work that cannot be done alone.

References

Bynum, Caroline Walker. *The Resurrection of the Body in Western Christianity, 200–1336*. Lectures on the History of Religions; New Ser., No. 15. New York: Columbia University Press, 1995.

Foster, Charles R. *Educating Clergy: Teaching Practices and the Pastoral Imagination*. 1st ed. San Francisco: Jossey-Bass, 2006.

Ghosh, S.K. "Human Cadaveric Dissection: A Historical Account from Ancient Greece to the Modern Era." *Anatomy & Cell Biology* 48, no. 3 (2015): 153–69.

Gill-Austern, B.L. "Rediscovering Hidden Treasures for Pastoral Care." *Pastoral Psychology* 43 (1995): 233–53.

---

[17] Emmanuel Levinas, "Ideology and Idealism," in *The Levinas Reader*, ed. Seán Hand (Oxford: Basil Blackwell, 2002), 247.
[18] Ibid.

Jotterand, F. "The Hippocratic Oath and Contemporary Medicine: Dialectic between Past Ideals and Present Reality?" *Journal of Medical Philosophy* 30, no. 1 (2005): 107–28.

Levin, Jeffrey S. *Religion and Medicine: A History of the Encounter between Humanity's Two Greatest Institutions*. New York: Oxford University Press, 2020.

Levinas, Emmanuel. "Ideology and Idealism." In *The Levinas Reader*, edited by Seán Hand, 235–48. Oxford: Basil Blackwell, 2002.

Lévinas, Emmanuel, and Philippe Nemo. *Ethics and Infinity*. 1st ed. Pittsburgh: Duquesne University Press, 1985.

May, William F. *The Physician's Covenant: Images of the Healer in Medical Ethics*. 2nd ed. Lexington, KY: Westminster John Knox Press, 2000.

Norman, Kathryn E. "This Is My Body." *Journal of the American Medical Association* 320, no. 5 (2018): 441–2.

Vesalius, Andreas. *On the Fabric of the Human Body in Seven Books*. [in Content in Latin]. Basel, Switzerland: Joannes Oporinus, 1555.

Volf, Miroslav, Matthew Croasmun, and Ryan McAnnally-Linz. *Life Worth Living: A Guide to What Matters Most*. New York: The Open Field/Penguin Life, 2023.

3
The Ages of Medicine and Faith

Chapter Outline

Care and Cure: Age of the Priest/Physician	35
Healing and Christianity	37
The World Before Ours: Ptolemaic Medicine	45
Ptolemaic Cosmology and Medicine and Faith	49
The Changing Modes of Medicine	52
Slow Medicine and Fast Medicine	58

The historical relation of medicine and faith has never been static, since both sides of the relation have changed and developed. Prior modes of interaction have left their marks on our contemporary setting, so in this chapter we will briefly consider three reference points of particular importance: the gospel healing miracles, the Ptolemaic cosmological framework that shaped the relation of medicine and religion in the west for the better part of 2,000 years, and the stages of modern medicine.

Care and Cure: Age of the Priest/Physician

Medicine has always been a mix of care and treatment, both support for the person and the body that are afflicted as well as treatment aimed at what particularly ails that person. Care enhances the natural underlying processes (like diet, activity, community, sleep) that affect health. Treatment alters the actual course of the illness, hopefully ameliorating or curing it, though possibly aggravating the condition or creating new problems. For most of history, it was hard to sharply distinguish care from treatment. Many of the things offered as treatment (bloodletting, purgatives) had little direct effect on the cause of the illness and actually undermined healthy natural processes. In scientific hindsight, some treatments derived from practical wisdom passed down in tradition were likely beneficial (for instance, the consumption of herbs or plants from which contemporary drugs have later been derived).

In ages where most healthy people lived on the edge of resource sufficiency, the difference between fighting off an illness or injury and succumbing to it could often come down to access to food, water, and shelter, and, perhaps most importantly, to the social companionship required for these. Medical "experts" could primarily offer descriptive knowledge, commentary, and companionship to those who were sick. Based on prior observation, such a person might diagnose (i.e., recognize) what afflicted you, might provide a prognosis predicting its likely course, but could rarely do anything to decisively change the underlying dynamics of the disease. The role of such a person was not clearly distinct from that of a religious leader or a folk healer. Medical anthropology suggests that most human cultures have featured healers spanning a spectrum that ran from exorcist-priest-magician to folkloric technician, from shamans to tooth pullers.[1] Such practices and practitioners coexisted, and certainly did not fall out into opposing camps.

Even in a primarily "medical" mode, causes and treatments were often associated with what we would categorize as religious issues: demonic possession or physical effects of moral or spiritual failings. A healer might diagnose and respond to spiritual, moral, or emotional states—despair, guilt, anxiety—with treatments that seem more biological in nature (ointments, particular foods, or drinks). And they might respond to bodily symptoms with the administration of more "religious" remedies: sacramental activities, rituals, asceticism. No clear demarcation set off spiritual concerns from purely physical ones. For most of the history of medicine, certainly down

---

[1] Lawrence Eugene Sullivan, *Healing and Restoring: Health and Medicine in the World's Religious Traditions* (New York; London: Macmillan; Collier Macmillan, 1989).

into the nineteenth century, the role of doctor and that of priest broadly overlapped.

The sharp divergence of medicine and religion is a recent phenomenon. That separation, led by a certain reductive intensity of focus in medicine, has been enormously fruitful for human health. At the same time, we have more and more begun to recognize the failures of this approach to reckon with the significance of things excluded by that very focus: the social determinants of health, the environmental factors in disease, the epigenetic impact of human behavior on our own biology, mind-body feedback. In other words, the wider nexus that was methodologically excluded in modern medicine (the better to focus on the intricate complexity of our physical biology) but was so integral to the pre-modern world, re-emerges as an important part of the medical picture.

The historical departure point was one in which two modes of healing, the spiritual and the biological, belonged to the same spectrum. Even the most radical forms of spiritual transformation implied a physical/medical dimension, and even the most technical medical interventions had an explicitly spiritual context. This was simply a feature of the cosmologies that people inhabited. Our ancestors commonly assumed human physical bodies were in some measure tuned to or microcosms of the wider cosmic and natural world. Their world integrated what we would call religious and spiritual assumptions into what we would call its science and technologies. This nexus was the premise not only of medical practices but of religious, social and political ones as well. What ails us and restores us is bound up with what things mean, where we come from, and how we are to live.

"Faith healing" conjures up images of ministers casting out demons or confidently calling on God to instantly restore a paralyzed person or remove their cancer. It suggests the polar opposite of contemporary medicine, a spiritual approach that is indifferent to or aggressively opposed to instrumental or biological treatment. But this perceived opposition is partly based on the illusion that a "faith only" approach has been the characteristic religious approach to healing in the past, or is the most characteristic one now.

Healing and Christianity

Such exclusionary insistence has never been the predominant approach to healing in Christianity. Appeal to divine healing is always part of the Christian response to illness and disability. What supportive care (hydration, food, rest) is to medical prescriptions—the assumed base line for all therapeutic regimes—prayer, petition, and community are to spiritual ones. Such things need not be and rarely are the entire story, but they are always commended. Likewise, in its very nature faith affirms the possibility of healing, even miraculous physical healing, that goes beyond what any medical treatment might expect.

Between this "nothing less than" reliance on divine sustenance, personal spirituality, and community ritual and support, and the "over and above" hope of divine-human synergy that exceeds the scope of normal medical hope, is the broad realm where religion concretely interacts with medicine. This zone has obviously changed as medicine itself has changed. Christians through the ages had no principled commitment to eschew medical treatments in favor of ecclesial ones alone. Indeed, Christian institutions often conceived, adopted, and fostered medical treatments as part of their own vocations. Hospitals in the Western world originated in the hostels, infirmaries, and poor shelters of monasteries or dioceses.[2] Some Christian and Christian-derived groups do maintain that faith treatments should be the default approach. And it remains sadly true that in much of the world lack of access to medical care means that religious and traditional resources remain a default resort of the poor, as they do for the desperate ones for whom scientific medicine has proved inadequate. The widespread Christian sponsorship of medical services reflects the common belief that divine healing moves most often in concert with the "secondary causes" of medical modalities, as support and enhancement, and only rarely stands out beyond or above them.

The mandate to pursue physical healing as part of Christian life goes to the very root: the healings by Jesus (and by others in his name) in the New Testament scriptures. That Jesus healed people is probably one of the most historically grounded and least distinctive things about him, considered as a first-century charismatic spiritual leader. It would have been an expectation for a teacher with a claim to divine authority as much as it would have been for a physician with a claim to medical wisdom. And just as the practices of the "physicians" of that time include much to us that looks religious, so we

---

[2] Guenter B. Risse, *Mending Bodies, Saving Souls: A History of Hospitals* (New York: Oxford University Press, 1999).

can see that the physical cures attributed to Jesus are presented as healings of the person, as much as curing of their disease.

One thing the texts illustrate is the firm conviction, widespread in most religions, that there is a connection between spiritual truth and physical well-being. "Salvation" is a word whose roots in Latin and Greek both point to deliverance from death, physical healing, and well-being. Religious redemption is a deeper, wider form of well-being, one for which physical health is both a metaphor and a partial realization. The healing miracles of Jesus reflect this.

Those healing events manifest compassion for the physical suffering of the persons involved, but they are also meant by Jesus as signs of the "kingdom of God." Which means they are meant to show that physical illness and suffering were not the divine plan for creation and that the fulfillment of that plan would include their abolition. For later Christians, the mandate to care for and heal the sick seems to have required nothing more than the example set by Jesus and the commandments given by him in the gospels. This was powerfully reinforced by belief in the *bodily* resurrection of Jesus. Since the beginning of the tradition, Christian writers have stretched medical terms to speak of resurrection as a comprehensive healing of human nature, not through the liberation of spirit from matter, but through the infusion of a new kind life which renders bodies "incorruptible," no longer subject to their failings. Those who hoped their bodies would be raised as Jesus' was had an additional reason to care for their bodies and value them.

Christian tradition developed a reading of scripture and the events in scripture that found four overlapping meanings in the same text: a literal, a moral, an allegorical, and a mystical meaning. According to the literal sense, an account of Jesus healing a visually impaired person refers to an actual encounter, a physical or medical change for that person. According to the moral sense, the teaching of the text is that as Jesus cared for people's physical infirmities, so should disciples of Jesus do the same. The moral teaching is an imperative to care for the sick: the *means* of that caring may be medical or spiritual or both. According to the allegorical sense, the recovery of sight signifies not a medical event but an awakening to a new outlook, a conversion of spirit. We are all people in need of this transformation, and "was blind but now I see" is not the story of a person with a particular ophthalmological need, but a diagnosis that applies to all of us, quite apart from our physical health. The mystical sense interprets scripture not for what it tells us about past events, or what it teaches us for current activity, but for what it points to as a final, eschatological hope. This healing story foretells that in the final realization of the divine plan we will all perceive each other and God with a new immediacy: "For now we see in a mirror, dimly, but then we will see face to face."[3]

Gospel writers often focus less on what we would call the medical miracle and more on spiritual lessons about forgiveness, reconciliation, or the Kingdom of God. For instance, in Mk 2:3-12, a paralyzed man is lowered through an opening his friends have dug in a roof, to present him before Jesus. Jesus says to the obviously disabled man, "Son, your sins are forgiven." There are skeptics in the crowd who ask, quite justly, "Why does this fellow speak in this way? It is blasphemy! Who can forgive sins but God alone?" Jesus responds, "Why do you raise such questions in your hearts? Which is easier, to say to the paralytic, 'Your sins are forgiven,' or to say, 'Stand up and take your mat and walk'? But so that you may know that the Son of Man has authority on earth to forgive sins"—he said to the paralytic—"I say to you, stand up, take your mat and go to your home." The man then does exactly that. It seems that Jesus' primary work here is to forgive the sins of the man, rather than physically heal him. The physical healing is attached as a kind of certification to the overcoming of an affliction possibly even more permanent than paralysis: guilt and estrangement.

In this case, we have the peculiar details about the group who sought care for their friend, even by the extreme measure of lowering him through the roof. Their faith and hope were directed toward Jesus, but it was expressed through a vicarious act of solidarity with their friend. The stories not only illustrate Jesus' stature and the reality of divine power but stress an orientation of trust and mutual support that is the optimal openness to that grace. In this case, the act of faith was not from the paralyzed man, but rather from his friends. They cared for him enough and believed in Jesus enough to come through the roof. It is the supportive web of community that makes the healing possible.

A major aspect of the suffering entailed by a disease is precisely the social ostracism and isolation associated with it, and a key aspect of the healing is the restoration to relation and participation. In the Gospel of Luke, there is a man afflicted with leprosy, a horribly disfiguring skin infection (Lk. 5:12-16). We know today that leprosy is caused by a mycobacterium, a cousin to tuberculosis, that infects the nerves and deadens them, which leads to complicated vascular compromise and susceptibility to infection. The effects

---

[3] 1 Corinthians 13:12.

of leprosy—the bacteriological affliction—have no medical cure. Once the nerves die, they cannot be revived. The long-term effect of smoldering infections and micro-traumas is significant mutilation of the face and limbs. There were also other skin conditions that caused significant disfigurement clustered in the category of leprosy. In the ancient world, people with leprosy were excluded from communal and religious life. They were the ultimate outsiders. Leprosy cut across social class and gender. If you had leprosy, you were estranged from religious and communal life. You were also estranged from God. The medical term has become a social one in our culture, and "treating someone like a leper" signifies a category of social affliction all its own, without any need for a medical diagnosis.

A leper approaches Jesus, "Lord, if you choose, you can make me clean." The word "clean" points to more than just the physical disfigurement of leprosy, but refers to the social impurity and religious condemnation associated with it. Jesus stretches out his hand, touches him, and says, "I do choose. Be made clean." The touch is itself a cure, a reversal of the isolation and social condemnation enforced by physical distance. Luke writes that the leprosy is immediately cured, but the story is not over. Jesus tells the man, "Go . . . and show yourself to the priest, and, as Moses commanded, make an offering for your cleansing, for a testimony to them." This, in turn, would restore the man to a place in his community. The common theme to all these stories is the work of reconciliation. A person with leprosy can now mix with others and worship; the paralyzed man takes up his mat and is restored to his community.

When we discuss these healing stories with a mixture of ministry students and those from medical fields, religious people and secular people, the conversation rarely runs aground on flat conflict over their plausibility. The mechanics of healing in the texts is a kind of blank space, frankly ascribed to a mysterious divine source. Almost everything that a medical account would regard as directly relevant is missing. Instead, we learn a great deal about the social, religious, and moral environment of the person, their illness, and the resulting changes associated with healing. It is a mirror image of a medical account, which specifies the specific bacteria implicated in an infection and the drug whose mechanism has been found to most effectively eradicate it, or specifies a mineral deficiency and the pathway by which this leads to a particular biological malfunction. In these medical accounts, everything is (ideally, though rarely actually) accounted for at a physical level, but almost nothing is accounted for in all the dimensions detailed in the healing stories. We often speak of and experience medical cures as miraculous, when in fact their mechanism may be clearly understood: it is their wider meaning and impact in our lives that we indicate with the word. On the other hand, there are forms of brokenness, ostracism, and pain that persist even in medical success.

This imbalance in focus between the medical and the spiritual accounts means that when we search for medical explanations of the healing miracles we gravitate toward more contextual or psychosomatic approaches. Perhaps the person possessed by demons suffered from a mental illness, for which social acceptance was a mitigating factor. Perhaps the paralysis that was cured was a psychological symptom of past trauma that religious absolution unlocked. The medical model of healing offers paths to recovered function: the tumor removed, the electrolytes normalized. A spiritual model offers reconciliation and social renewal, induces psychological and even biophysical plasticity. It deals as much in the relief of suffering and the support of hope as it does in physical capacities.

Today, as in biblical times, people often associate medical ills with moral and spiritual ones. The idea that disease is a divine punishment for wrongdoing answers the otherwise opaque question of why it afflicts one person and not another. Many of the healing miracles have this assumed relation between physical disease and someone's moral or religious status as a clear backdrop. When Jesus heals a man born blind, the people ask "Who sinned, the man born blind or his parents?"[4] Jesus rejects the assumptions of his interrogators that physical affliction follows this kind of moral causation. God desires both to forgive sin and to restore bodies.

In Jesus' time, people believed that a moral or religious taint in someone could attract disease, that we were blamable for individually or corporately compromising the moral and religious immunity systems that protected us. So healing extended both to bodies and to our spiritual and communal relations. There are modern parallels to these healing stories. We judge others in their illness in ways subtle and overt. While ostracizing lepers seems archaic and cruel, our world is no stranger to the same impulse. Today, we may indict or exclude people for their diet and life choices, for an inherited defect in their personal genome, or even for their health care decisions.

Take the neighbor with newly diagnosed lung cancer. The first question we ask is, "How much did she smoke?" Take the family member who suffers

---

[4] John 9:2-12.

a car accident. "How fast was he driving?" We cast blame. We think less of those who suffer illness. We have been particularly cruel to those who suffer with HIV, particularly during the 1980s when we understood less about it. Religious perspectives did much to support that cruelty. "With whom did she have sex?" "Did he share needles?" The suffering of the illness was multiplied by the social judgements. The person with HIV now lives nearly as long as those without the infection. But the stigma still lingers.

The most toxic interpretation of these biblical passages over the years has turned the association of faith with cure into a negative conclusion: a lack of healing flows from a lack of faith. If you do not recover, despite your prayers and those of others, then there must be something lacking in the faith behind them. We have seen that prayer is the universal Christian response to illness, a "nothing less" that appears to be the ultimate noninvasive treatment. But prayer, under certain assumptions can also have side effects, and in such cases the side effect is despair and guilt.

When Jesus heals a boy with epilepsy after his disciples cannot, they ask him why they failed, and he answers, "Because of your little faith. For truly I tell you, if you have faith the size of a mustard seed, you will say to this mountain, 'Move from here to there,' and it will move; and nothing will be impossible for you."[5] Nothing is impossible! If so, then every painful and tragic outcome is a spiritual failure and every medical intervention is an admission of religious defeat.

Put this baldly, we can see not only that Christians have rarely drawn this conclusion but that the scriptures themselves do not run in this direction. We get a different indication from Jesus' own prayer before his death, asking God, "if it is possible, let this cup pass from me; yet not what I want but what you want."[6] The apostle Paul famously suffered from an unspecified physical affliction (that he called the "thorn in his flesh") which he did not attribute to a failing in his faith, but accepted as a trial to strengthen him.[7] When Christians are exhorted to visit the sick, they are not sent to reproach them for not getting better.

Healing has at least four levels we discussed earlier: a literal one at the level of physical cure, a moral one at the level of altered behavior and social reconciliation, an allegorical one in a transformation of meaning or self-

---

[5] Matthew 17:20.
[6] Matthew 26:39.
[7] 2 Corinthians 12:7.

understanding, and a mystical one regarding our future hope. This then means also that the miracle of healing can take any of these forms. A chaplain in an oncology unit found that many of her patients and their families expressed a hope for a miracle. When she asked them "what does a miracle look like for you?" she was somewhat surprised by the answers. For one it would be for their spouse to regain consciousness and lucidity long enough to say good bye. For another it was if they found a lessening of the chronic pain that remained after successful treatment for their tumor. Some found a reconciliation between estranged family members or friends in midst of the trial of illness to be a miracle.

The "mountain" in question need not be a biological one though it may involve a dimension of the physical. It may appear quite impossible from the best medical judgment that someone will resist their cancer long enough to see their grandchild born, and yet they do. Sometimes a perfectly prosaic instance of medical cure has behind it a more complicated miracle. A Christian doctor and nurse team in Alabama were told by all they consulted that their dream to provide no-cost health care to the uninsured poor without any government support could not possibly work. But their clinic now cares for 25,000 patients.[8] People whose lives are saved or changed there by what is scientifically prosaic medical care have been in a real sense healed by faith. The faith that moves mountains is a reality, but it is a gift and not a guarantee.

In the healing stories, divine power is never directly presented as a competitor with or as excluding any medical type of healing. There is a passing reference in the account of the healing of a woman with a uterine hemorrhage, noting that she had consulted "many physicians" and her condition had only become worse.[9] But this only explains her desperation and does not disparage any aid those physicians might render. The horizon of Jesus' healing activity is set by a condition where medical healing is out of the question.

The simplest illustration of this is the story of the raising of Lazarus.[10] Jesus' close friend Lazarus has died and been two days in the tomb when Jesus is summoned, weeping, to the grave and calls out "Lazarus, come forth." Upon which Lazarus rises in his burial garments and resumes his life.

---

[8] G. Scott Morris and Jim Wallis, *Care: How People of Faith Can Respond to Our Broken Health System* (Grand Rapids, MI: Eerdmans, William B. Publishing Company, 2022), 129.
[9] Mark 5:24-34; Luke 8:42-48.
[10] John 11:17-44

There are many fascinating aspects to this text, but for our purpose the simplest is the most important. This miracle strikes us as the most extreme sort—not the unexpected recovery from illness but the very reversal of death, as if one had successfully performed CPR two days after the fact. But it is notable for what it does not achieve.

Whatever infirmity killed Lazarus is (temporarily) overcome. But Lazarus will die again, definitively, as all people will, including those healed by Jesus, including Jesus himself. The story of the raising of Lazarus leads into the passion narrative of Jesus' death and resurrection (his resuscitation of Lazarus is given as one of the things that prompts others to plot his death), which constitutes the remainder of the Gospel of John. This juxtaposition makes a clear point. All medical healings, even divinely instituted ones, have the same limits. They are restoration or even reversal. Resurrection is something quite different. It is life beyond death, no longer subject to its power or prospect. The animating origin of the church was not the conviction that Lazarus or Jesus had been reprieved from death for a few years, but belief in an event of an entirely different order. The implication was not that any such earthly healings were of no account by comparison with that hope, but that they found a new meaning as shadows and prefigurations of it.

The World Before Ours: Ptolemaic Medicine

We stand too close to our own context for the relation of medicine with religion to imagine it otherwise. For that reason, it is worthwhile to briefly visit the cosmological world that preceded ours, with its quite different assumptions about that relation. We said earlier that faith and medicine have freely intertwined in history, particularly in what we called the zone in between the supportive spiritual resources always deployed in illness and the "over and beyond" appeal to unmediated divine action. In the Western world, from the time of the Greeks and the Romans, this largely amicable juxtaposition of medical labors and spiritual aspirations was represented by treatment focused in the temple on one hand and treatment focused on an individual physician on the other.

In the ancient Greek world, if you were sick, you likely would consult with local folkloric wise persons as well as a priest of Asclepius, the healing god.[11] The priest would hear your concerns, and then invite you to spend the night in their temple, the Asclepion. Snakes would be slithering about the site as special mascots because the shedding of their skins was a symbol of renewal and new life. The temple would also have stone stellae with testimony of the extraordinary recoveries that had occurred there. In the morning, you would consult with the priest about your dreams. Interpretation of dreams would be one means to identify a cure. Likely, you would be prescribed purgatives or cathartics, potions for your skin, or bloodletting.

Alternatively or additionally, you might consult with a physician, a "professional" more than a priest, with special learning and training. The Hippocratic tradition of medicine, as distinct from divine healing (a distinction foreign to those in this tradition themselves), was the basis on which all Jewish, Christian, and Islamic medicine developed. The great Islamic and Jewish figures Avicenna and Maimonides were famed in their lifetimes as much as physicians as religious scholars. And the medicine they practiced had been pioneered by the paragon of the Hippocratic tradition, the second-century CE physician, Galen.[12] He hailed from Pergamum, site of a grand shrine to Asclepius, association with which was part of his mystique. The most renowned doctor of his day, who cared personally for Roman emperors, Galen understood himself equally to be a philosopher. His writings comprise as much as half of the extant Greek manuscripts from the ancient world, indicating that such medical work weighed at least as much on the scales of literate esteem as that of those still famous to us, like Plato and Aristotle. Those writings on anatomy and disease formed the core curriculum of medical schools for over 1,000 years. An acute observer, who dissected animals though not humans, Galen's textual authority became so great that it inhibited any empirical correction until the sixteenth century.

The world in which Galenic medicine fit was the Ptolemaic universe, a cosmology that predated him and would endure to the time of Copernicus. By stepping back to view this wider perspective, one can appreciate a feature of his medicine (and indeed also of the religious "temple" medicine of the same time) that is not readily apparent up close: its extraordinary coherence

---

[11] For the paragraph that follows, see Trevor Curnow, "The Cult of Asclepius: Its Origins and Early Development," *Bulletin of the John Rylands Library (2014)* 89 (2013): 67–83.

[12] On Galen, see Erwin H. Ackerknecht, *A Short History of Medicine*, Revised and expanded ed. (Baltimore, MD: Johns Hopkins University Press, 2016), 73–8.

or holism. The terms by which healer and healed understood sickness were continuous with those by which one understood all other matters, from the astronomical and agricultural to the spiritual and metaphysical. This provided a kind of intelligibility and systemic support that is hard for us to imagine.

In the Ptolemaic cosmology, the earth stood as a small speck in the middle of a vast space.[13] The orbit of the moon marked a boundary line, separating the astronomical realm above (where unchanging perfection was the rule) from the mutable and grossly material realm below. The moon marked not just a geographical border, but an evaluative one. The ancients are much derided by their modern successors for the egocentric confidence with which they placed the earth at the center of their universe. But in their universe the center was the absolutely worst place to be. It was the cellar, the pits, the place far below the eternal heavens, the place where imperfect forms of spirit went to spoil, as it were, and spawn physical things.

The planets revolved on their eternal spheres, and the stars revolved together on one majestic outer sphere. In the sublunar realm, the four constituent material elements (earth, water, air, and fire) naturally occupied concentric spheres: earth at the center, water around the earth, air around the water, and fire above the air just under the moon's orbit. These elements had become mixed, in some measure dislodged from their natural places, to form all the composite forms of matter we know. Trees, for instance, have mixed fire, air, water, and earth through the natural processes of their growth. When a piece of wood is burned, we see these elements released and returned to their natural places—the trapped bits of fire leaping upward as flame, air rising as smoke, water as steam or smoke, and earth falling back as ash to its place at the center. Motion was largely explained by this idea of natural place. Things made of earth return to their natural place at the center (i.e., fall) when not constrained. Rain falls from the sky because water seeks its natural sphere around the earth. Things of composite nature have correspondingly complex characters.

Human health, illness, and medicine were understood within this same cosmological scheme. One of the hallmarks of Galenic medicine was the

---

[13]For a lovely concise description of this cosmology and the features discussed here, see C.S. Lewis, *The Discarded Image: An Introduction to Medieval and Renaissance Literature* (Cambridge: Cambridge University Press, 1967).

extension of that cosmology into a "humoral" system.[14] He amplified Hippocrates' theory that disease was caused by an imbalance of four substances or "humors" in the human body: black bile, yellow bile, phlegm, and blood. Each humor had its own qualities, and was associated with (primarily composed of) one of the four basic elements. Black bile was cold and wet, made mainly of earth and associated with the autumn season. If you had an abundance of black bile in your body, you would suffer from depression, melancholia, from *melana* which means black, and *chole* which is bile. In contrast, yellow bile had properties of hot and dry, was rich with the element fire and associated with the summer season. A person with an abundance of yellow bile would be choleric in nature, ambitious, angry, and short-tempered. Phlegm was cold and wet, full of water and paired with the winter season. Phlegmatic people tend to be relaxed, quiet, calm, and observant. Blood is primarily made of the element air and associated with springtime. A preponderance of blood—a sanguine person—makes one sociable, charismatic, and outgoing. As we can see, the balance or flux in the elements was seen as the "scientific" cause in things as diverse as human personality traits and the turn of nature's seasons.

It is hard to quantify the significance for patients of the intelligibility of their disease and treatment, by which I mean the degree to which these make intuitive sense to them. In this cosmology, the medical world is profoundly integrated into the wider one, into the spiritual, moral, and natural landscape. From such a perspective, astronomy was an important component of medicine. The spheres of the individual planets revolved and transmitted an influence down the interlocking spheres below, affecting life on earth. Each planet was associated with a different humor and could influence your health, for instance by its dominant celestial position in the zodiac at the time of your birth. This has come down to us in the language of astrology.

So interlocked are these layers of meaning that it is often hard to know what to count as religion and what as science in our terms. Christian peasants might, like their pagan neighbors, bury metal plates with planetary symbols in their fields. Was this a religious ritual or scientific agricultural practice? One Christian bishop, presented with this question, decided it was acceptable as best-practice husbandry, but advised his parishioners not to accompany

---

[14] Content in the following paragraph is drawn from John M. Riddle, "Theory and Practice in Medieval Medicine," in *Viator Medieval and Renaissance Studies: Volume 5 (1974)* (Berkeley: University of California Press, 2023), 161–88.

the burial with any ritual or invocation in the name of the planet. That would be to treat the planet too much like a god. Christians adopted a similar attitude toward the Galenic medicine that they employed.

The fact that a remedy has intuitive appeal to us proves nothing about its biological efficacy. But we understand that what makes sense to us as helpful tends for that reason to actually help us more than it otherwise would. Contemporary medicine would call this an enhanced placebo effect, attached to treatments whose logic seems self-evident to the recipient. And this dimension goes deep in the Ptolemaic/Galenic medical world. The four elements and their balances were seen as operative in all spheres. Cures for illnesses were aimed at rebalancing the four humors. For fevers, one of the most tried remedies was bloodletting. Fevers were due to an abundance of wetness and heat—blood. Thus, the obvious course would be to relieve the body of this imbalance by bloodletting. Different foods, because of their varied compositions, were thought of as remedies or antidotes for unhealthy imbalances. For example, lavender and lemon balm were used to treat melancholia, the buildup of black bile. These herbs were thought to incite warmth and moisture and so counteract the buildup of cold and dry black bile.

Our modern cosmology has grand unifying features, as for instance in the structure of DNA that underlies all living things. The insights it offers provide unparalleled therapeutic power for medicine. But these unities are highly abstract and intellectual. They do not have the immediacy of those in the Ptolemaic world, nor do they provide a bridge of intelligibility uniting the popular with the expert. And they do not imbue nature with the same intuitive power for evaluative and personal meaning.

Ptolemaic Cosmology and Medicine and Faith

The Ptolemaic and Galenic world is one that Jews, Christians, and Muslims inherited. They had no significant role in creating it. In many respects, they accepted it as the consensual "science" of their time, shared without regard to religion, and they adapted theological interpretation to this context. For instance, much imagery that we take to be intrinsically Christian in fact represents an accommodation of biblical material to this inherited cosmological setting. That Christians came to teach that there were nine ranks or orders of angels comes not from a biblical model but from the Ptolemaic fact that there are nine planets thought to be arranged in a hierarchical order. The angel Gabriel, who came to communicate with Mary the mother of Jesus was said to be an archangel, a relatively low rank among the nine. Why was this so? Because angels had to remain near to their proper sphere in the heavens, and this message would have been transmitted from one closer to the highest heaven to one further down and so on until it reached an angel who could, as it were, breathe in the atmosphere below the moon.

Christians did not have an alternative cosmology to replace the one around them and, as the illustration suggests, they tended to assimilate to it. But at certain key points, they did break with Ptolemaic assumptions, points with important implications for medicine. For instance, the Ptolemaic universe embodies an evaluative belief, an assumption that the center of the cosmos is its worst location, that matter is intrinsically inferior to spirit, that the truest divinity is least connected to the material world and resides at the furthest remove from it. In contrast with this, Christians followed Jews in affirming a creator God, whose material creation was intrinsically good. Further, they believed that this God had become incarnate; that is, had become one of the mutable, material creatures. Through this incarnation, Christians further believed, humans would be raised bodily from the dead. Taken together, these convictions amounted to a major revaluation of the character of bodily health.

Christians are often associated with ascetic and world-denying dimensions of spirituality, where material concerns are subordinated to the pursuit of spiritual ones. This has been a very real feature of Christian practice, but the idea that Christians cared only for the life of the spirit and denigrated the life of the body is misleading at best. That aspect of spirituality did not represent something peculiarly Christian, but a continuity with the cultural environment, an outlook that seemed obvious to surrounding (and competing) religious and philosophical traditions.

Christians might sometimes claim to excel others in what was a common aspiration to suppress the dominance of our bodily impulses and interests. That aspiration was "baked in" to the very structure of the inherited cosmology we have described. The peculiarity in biblical perspectives was found elsewhere, in this idea that the material world itself, *as bodily and mutable,* had an eternal value and future. This was reflected both in a retrospective belief in an Edenic state of nature and humanity, where the material created world had come from God's hand as good, and a prospective hope for a "new heaven and earth" including resurrected bodies. The Christian message can devolve into "pie in the sky by and by," but that reality should not obscure the dramatic significance of its root insistence that it is the bodily, material world as a whole that has an ultimate destiny and is the subject of healing. That outlook situated normal medicine as a kind of interim response to a human state (bodily susceptibility to injury and disease) that was not itself final.

"Christian medicine," if we may call it that, combined the medicine shared by all who lived in that assumed, enchanted cosmos with this different idiom of biblical perspective. The provision of medical care became a primary function of the church. Hospitals and hospices took their name and their vocation from a root concern for hospitality. They were places of shelter and care (including medical care), and those they sheltered were understood first as guests more than patients. In French, hospitals, particularly those for the poor, are called *hôtel de dieu*, God's hostel or hotel.

These facilities, often connected with monasteries, were an explicit melding of church and clinic. In places like Beaune, France, one can still see the shape this took. In a long, open space, individual beds were lined against the walls where the patients could be cared for easily by the staff. This ward was at the same time a sanctuary, for at one end stood an altar at which services would be celebrated, with all those bedridden present and participating.

One of the great works of late medieval art belongs to just such a setting. It is the famous Isenheim altarpiece.[15] Now in a museum, it originally stood in a church built alongside a hospital. The clinic in question treated large numbers of persons with what was then called Saint Anthony's fire, because it was believed to have been an affliction suffered by the saint. This is now supposed to be ergotism, caused by eating rye grain contaminated with a fungus.

Painful and unsightly skin sores were a central symptom of the disease. And what is so striking about the altarpiece is that those sores, which also are very similar to those contracted in some forms of plague, have been

---

[15] Andrée Hayum, *The Isenheim Altarpiece: God's Medicine and the Painter's Vision*, Princeton Essays on the Arts (Princeton, NJ: Princeton University Press, 1989); Michael Schubert, *The Isenheim Altarpiece: History—Interpretation—Background*, English ed. (Hudson Stuttgart: SteinerBooks; SchneiderEditionen, 2017).

replicated not only in the scenes of St. Anthony's suffering, but on the body of the crucified Jesus.

In the communal wards, patients were cared for with the best medical means then conceivable, the Galenic approach inherited from pre-Christian sources. In the case of these patients, this meant little more than a few ointments and amputation of gangrenous limbs. At the same time, they were constantly overseen with reminders that their suffering was shared and understood by their savior. They were cared for physically, but also encompassed in a wider community of solidarity and hope. The altarpiece was the setting for the regular representation in worship of the general Christian story of death and resurrection, but that story's artistic representation had been diagnostically particularized, we might say, to the condition of these patients.

In such settings, the structurally holistic setting for health and medicine in the Ptolemaic universe had been suffused with a specifically religious perspective that undergirded instrumental medical care and offered hope and meaning that went beyond it. Down to the present day, in Christian medical facilities, one can still see the outlines of that earlier unified vision, even while the medical care it partners with has changed in extraordinary ways.

There was something beautiful, consoling, and, to some extent, healing about this integration. But in terms of practical effect on the course of the disease or theoretical understanding of its nature, such a model was desperately weak. It would be transformed by the coming changes in the modes of medicine.

The Changing Modes of Medicine

The dominance of Galenic medicine began to recede in the sixteenth century. The Renaissance and the Reformation upended intellectual assumptions on many fronts and modern science started to emerge. Theology and medicine have often been swept up in a larger story of conflict between science and religion. Those who stress conflict rather than interaction maintain both science and medicine advanced by shaking off the domination of religious thought and turning instead toward a purely naturalistic commitment to empirical observation.

The simplistic version of this story has not survived historical examination.[16] Christian thought and institutions have inhibited and resisted scientific advances. They have just as often nurtured and stimulated them. At a deeper level, modern science was nurtured in late medieval thought and in a web of Christian assumptions. Two mutually informing assumptions in particular flowed from the biblical belief in creation. The first held that creation and nature have an internal intelligibility, because they are the work of an intelligent agent. The second held that this order was contingent, not deducible from first philosophical principles, because it was a free and personal act. These were crucial but hardly sufficient. As it happens, the turn among seventeenth-century Christians toward stressing the literal meaning in biblical texts (and using historical means to establish the text itself) as opposed to the multi-layered meanings of earlier exegesis, seems to have paralleled a similar approach to nature as having an empirically determinate character.[17] The "enchantment" of the Ptolemaic universe in which the spiritual and the material pervaded each other, began to unravel in both religious and scientific terms. The "book" of nature and the book of revelation were both to be searched for the *logos* animating them, but this was to be done, increasingly, by different methods.

In 1632, Galileo published his *Dialogue Concerning the Two Chief World Systems*, affirming the heliocentric universe Copernicus had privately advocated nearly seventy years before over the Ptolemaic model to which Jews and Christians had long adapted themselves. To modern sensibilities, this became a watershed moment that divided science and religion. Historians of science have long known the Galileo story itself is quite different from the caricature of factual observation versus superstitious dogma.[18] But what we

---

[16]The two books that popularized the conflict thesis in the American academic world were more polemic than scholarship, a point made tellingly in a video from the Dialogue on Science, Ethics, and Religion of the American Academy for the Advancement of Science. See The American Academy for the Advancement of Science, "Science and Religion: The Draper-White Conflict Thesis," https://youtu.be/ZLoZc5DIU9o. The books in question were Andrew Dickson White, *A History of the Warfare of Science with Theology in Christendom*, 2 vols. (New York; London: D. Appleton and company, 1932); John William Draper, *History of the Conflict between Religion and Science*, 5th ed. (New York: D. Appleton and company, 1875).
[17]See Peter Harrison, *The Bible, Protestantism, and the Rise of Natural Science* (Cambridge; New York: Cambridge University Press, 1998). See also Lesslie Newbigin, *Foolishness to the Greeks: The Gospel and Western Culture*, WCC Mission Series; No. 6 (Geneva: World Council of Churches, 1986). 70–1.
[18]See Derrick Peterson, "Galileo Again: Reevaluating Galileo's Conflict with the Church and Its Significance for Today," *Cultural Encounters: A Journal of Theology and Culture* 13, no. 1 (2017): 25–47.

might call the headline events of science-religion discussion for the coming centuries would be located in the realms of physics, cosmology, and geology (with questions like the age of the earth and the historicity of the biblical flood narrative). If one were to mount anti-religious arguments from science, physics would be the discipline from which to do it. By contrast, prior to Darwinian evolution, study of the living world was the favorite science of religious apologists, who saw the design and order there inexplicable apart from divine agency.

As theoretical institutional science emancipated itself from religious control, the practice of medicine retained more intimacy with ecclesial and spiritual life because it dealt with the concrete lives of its patients, because it continued to be set in hospitals and clinics organized by religious organizations, and because, though its discoveries might contradict Galenic authorities, they rarely conflicted in any explicit way with religious convictions. Nevertheless, the nature of the medicine with which religious thought and practice sought integration went through a series of dramatic transformations.

From the sixteenth to the twentieth centuries, Galenic medicine gave way to a succession of new models. The first we could call the hospital model. In the nineteenth century, Paris became the capital of western medicine.[19] Grand hospitals such as the La Salpêtrière for women, Les Enfants Trouvés and the L'Hôtel Dieu housed thousands of patients in long, open wards organized by symptom. The innovation was to move away from diagnosis as a one-on-one process between physician and patient, and to organize information through collective observation and analysis. Patients with dyspnea (shortness of breath) were in one ward, those with dropsy (fluid retention) in another. Rather than depending solely on a patient's self-reported history, physicians employed considerable new physical exam skills (observation, percussion, and palpation) as well as new instruments, like the stethoscope, in service of more systemic diagnosis and prognosis.

A feature of modern medical education emerged: patient rounds. The attending physician would preside over a group of learners and examine each patient in turn, highlighting physical exam findings and diagnosis. Young physicians came from around the world to learn from the great physicians of the Parisian hospitals, including Americans Benjamin Rush and Oliver

---

[19]Erwin Heinz Ackerknecht, *Medicine at the Paris Hospital, 1794-1848* (Baltimore, MD: Johns Hopkins Press, 1967); Ackerknecht, *A Short History of Medicine*, 146ff.

Wendell Homes Sr. A Parisian physician combined close observation with after-the-fact analysis through autopsies. But they offered little new in the way of therapeutics. The advance involved the collection of more detailed data and the better collation of that data to characterize specific diseases.

In the nineteenth century, the center of medicine moved from the Parisian wards into the laboratories of Berlin and Vienna.[20] Laboratory medicine replaced hospital medicine as the cutting edge of the discipline. The modern version of the physician-as-scientist emerged. The microscope emerged as the most emblematic tool. The body could be better understood through its chemical reactions and microscopic inhabitants.[21] Robert Koch, the most famous physician from this era, defined the method to isolate and identify microbial agents as causes of devastating human diseases, including anthrax, tuberculosis, and cholera.[22] Even without curative treatments, the identification of the causal agent in cholera, for instance, enabled a quantum leap in the prevention of illness through public health measures.

In the early twentieth century, the physician-scientist model became the archetype for medical training. In 1910, the Carnegie Foundation tasked Abraham Flexner with evaluating the quality of existing American medical schools.[23] The stakes were high. Those schools deemed unfit would be pressured to close. Those who fit the model would receive further funding. The paradigm of this new model was the Johns Hopkins medical school. Schools were required to have access both to patients and laboratories. Flexner recommended two years of basic sciences to provide students a foundation of pathophysiology, microbiology, and biochemistry, followed by two years of clinical training. This has remained the standard medical school curriculum for some one hundred years, and has only recently begun to shift. The Flexner model lifted the practice of medicine from that of a trade, largely learned by apprenticeship, to a respected profession with a unified methodology. This was a major frame-shift.

Initially, the fruit of the Johns Hopkins method was not new treatments, as these had not yet been discovered. It was subtraction, not addition. Sir

---

[20]See Chapters Fourteen and Fifteen in *A Short History of Medicine*.
[21]P.J. Ramberg, "The Death of Vitalism and the Birth of Organic Chemistry: Wohler's Urea Synthesis and the Disciplinary Identity of Organic Chemistry," *Ambix* 47, no. 3 (2000): 170–95.
[22]Steve M. Blevins and Michael S. Bronze, "Robert Koch and the 'Golden Age' of Bacteriology," *International Journal of Infectious Diseases* 14, no. 9 (2010): e744–e51.
[23]Kenneth M. Ludmerer, "Abraham Flexner and Medical Education," *Perspectives in Biology and Medicine* 54, no. 1 (2011): 8–16.

William Osler, perhaps the most famous doctor of his day, pointed out "that most of the remedies in common use were more likely to do harm than good."[24] Accurate diagnosis—determining what disease process was at work, what was its mechanism of effect in terms of the newly discovered chemical and microbal factors, and what was the likely natural course of the disease— became the gold standard of medical knowledge, even when nothing could be done to change the prognosis. But such knowledge was the precursor to effective therapies to come.

Pastoral care and theology reacted to this new model of medical care. Shortly after the standardization of medical education, theological education saw the birth of clinical pastoral education.[25] Medical schools had been in part modeled on the first graduate schools of any sort in the United States, theological seminaries. Such seminaries, like Andover in 1807, were founded on the assumption that an undergraduate degree was no longer sufficient preparation for ministry. Now, theological education adopted a version of medical rounds. Ministers and ministers in training were invited to go onto the clinical turf of the medical world—most typically general hospital wards, but also institutions caring for the mentally ill, rehabilitation and nursing homes—and to practice pastoral care on a clinical model. They would be assigned a segment of patients, carefully record their interactions, present their cases for peer feedback and receive supervision by senior chaplains and counselors. They would work as members of a care team alongside nurses and doctors, being instructed by them on the medical conditions of their patients, but also ministering to the medical care givers in their personal and spiritual needs. This program remains the most sustained educational framework for the interaction of religion and medicine.

After more than a century, is the physician-scientist model still the standard? Humanity has reaped the benefits of the physician-as-scientist approach to medical education. Life threatening diseases that the eighteenth century physician could only observe are now treated routinely. And yet, we live in a different age. How is memorizing the Krebs cycle important for septic shock? How is staining a slide important for treating a patient with tuberculosis? Clearly, a certain amount of science is important for medical training, but do we inflict fact overload upon our medical students at the

---

[24]Lewis Thomas, *The Youngest Science: Notes of a Medicine-Watcher* (Oxford; New York: Oxford University Press, 1985). 19–20.
[25]Stephen King, *Trust the Process: A History of Clinical Pastoral Education as Theological Education* (Lanham, MD: University Press of America 2007).

expense of clinical-based training? Is the model proposed by Flexner in 1910 still the model that we need today? Or is a new kind of holism needed?

In 2009, the accrediting council for US medical schools described six areas of core competency: fund of knowledge, patient care, practice-based learning and improvement, system-based practice, interpersonal and communication skills, and professionalism.[26] The physician-as-scientist model encompasses only a few of those six competencies—perhaps fund of knowledge and patient care—but barely addresses the others. All medical knowledge has a half-life. We no longer prescribe arsenic for syphilis or milkweed for pleurisy; but we do need physicians with a curiosity and discipline to continue their learning. We need innovators.

In 2017, the same accrediting council convened a task force to explore the changing landscape of medical education.[27] Members conducted more than 1,000 interviews with stake-holders nation-wide. They distilled three major forces that are shaping the medical profession: rapid democratization, increased commoditization, and advancing corporatization. Medical information is becoming increasingly available to all (democratization). As such, the delivery of medical care becomes indistinguishable from other products, with the primary difference point for units of medical care being price (commoditization). We see this in routine health care offerings in big box stores and bundled payments for surgical services. To manage all this, health care delivery has evolved into increasingly integrated, complex systems, such as regional hospital systems (corporatization).

The task force proposed future physicians should have the following attributes.[28] They should be *healers* who are able to make effective use of technology to enhance their healing relationship with patients. They should be *servant-leaders* who collaborate with others and prioritize the needs of others in decision-making. They should be *advocates* who promote patient-centered care and address social-determinants of health. They should be *team-members* who work and communicate with health care professionals toward effective coordination of patient care. The scientific substance of medicine—the ability to identify and treat conditions—here becomes almost a background assumption, and doctors are tasked with dauntingly

---

[26]Susan R. Swing et al., "Advancing Resident Assessment in Graduate Medical Education," *Journal of Graduate Medical Education* 1, no. 2 (2009): 278–86.
[27]For what follows, see John F. Duval et al., "Report of the Si2025 Task Force," *Journal of Graduate Medical Education* 9, no. 6s (2017): 11–57.
[28]Ibid.

comprehensive relational and managerial responsibilities. Is this "holism" dictated more by the need to negotiate an increasingly unwieldy health care system than by the outcomes most desired by patients and care givers?

We are entering a new age of medicine. To be a physician has become increasingly complex. Will we continue to fragment into more and more specialties: diagnosticians, proceduralists, coordinators, and specialized technicians?[29] Medicine is fraught with reconciling disparate, often contradictory, pieces of data and input from the perspectives of different specialties. Where is that synthesis to take place and who takes responsibility for it? The question arises for the cardiac surgeon who replaces heart valves, the geriatrician who conducts an end-of-life conversation with a family, and the primary care physician who navigates complicated drug-drug interactions. In this new age of medicine, are we called upon to reintegrate some of what was separated in earlier models?

Slow Medicine and Fast Medicine

As medicine evolved through the stages we have reviewed, premodern approaches were often regarded as completely outmoded, of interest to historians but of zero relevance to the practice of medicine. Victoria Sweet's book, *God's Hotel: A Doctor, a Hospital, and a Pilgrimage to the Heart of Medicine* reflects one doctor's experience of finding continuing relevance in that past and one of its figures. Sweet served as physician at the Laguna Honda hospital, a publicly funded rehabilitation facility in San Francisco serving many of its poorest citizens. She was, as the same time, pursuing a PhD in the history of medicine. She studied the work of Hildegard of Bingen, an abbess, medical writer and practitioner in twelfth-century Europe whose approach focused on mobilizing the body's healing processes.

Often overlooked in the intellectual tradition of the West, Hildegard was a polymath and mystic who made important contributions to medicine, music, and theology. One of the most influential women of the Middle Ages, she was prominent in the public sphere, rebuking popes and kings in preaching and writing. She was the composer of hymns and the recipient of

---

[29]Ohad Oren, Bernard J. Gersh, and Deepak L. Bhatt, "On the Pearls and Perils of Sub-Subspecialization," *The American Journal of Medicine* 133, no. 2 (2020): 158–9.

dramatic religious visions. [30] But she was equally prominent in her own time as a healer, the author of a medical handbook. [31] Hildegard stood in a millennium of continuity with Galenic medicine which she integrated with herbal folklore and theological teachings into her own theory of healing.[32]

The hymns she composed are still sung, nearly 1,000 years later. Perhaps her most famous is *O Virtus Sapientiae* which captures her mysticism: "O moving force of Wisdom, encircling the wheel of the cosmos, encompassing all that is, all that has life, in one vast circle." [33] If our world seeks engineering to fix the broken mechanics of our body, she pictured healers more like gardeners, tending the inner vitality in living things she called (in latin) their "*viriditas*." Literally, "greenness," *viriditas* was a quality of fecundity, the growth that sends out renewing shoots, an organism's inner knowledge of what it needs to flourish. Remove the impediments to healing, improve one's diet, rest, emotional health, and the body will strain to heal itself. In Hildegard's theology, the term bridged the biological and the spiritual. The *viriditas* in living things was a fount of physical health, but this was continuous with a spiritual "greening," in which moral virtue and faith made human life flourish. "The soul is the green life-force of the flesh."[34] Though other writers had used the term, Hildegard developed it in a unique way. For her, the divine spirit was the ultimate source of *viriditas*. All moral and spiritual gifts are "green with the greenness of the Holy Spirit."[35] She wrote "The Word is living, being, spirit, all verdant greening, all creativity . . . This

---

[30] See Sabina Flanagan, *Hildegard of Bingen, 1088-1179: A Visionary Life*, 2nd ed. (London; New York: Routledge, 1998); Victoria Sweet, *Rooted in the Earth, Rooted in the Sky: Hildegard of Bingen and Premodern Medicine*, Studies in Medieval History and Culture (New York: Routledge, 2006).

[31] See Margret Berger and Hildegard, *Hildegard of Bingen: On Natural Philosophy and Medicine: Selections from Cause Et Cure*, Library of Medieval Women (Cambridge; Rochester, NY: D.S. Brewer, 1999).

[32] The humoral theory still lives, albeit in a molecular form. There is increased interest in inflammatory cytokines such as interleukin 6 and tumor necrosis factor, which promote inflammation. Modern treatments for an over-abundance of these excessively heat-inducing proteins are cooling antibody blockers. During the Covid-19 pandemic, tocilizumab was used as an antibody which blocks interleukin 6. Infliximab, an antibody that blocks tumor necrosis factor, is used to treat a wide array of inflammatory diseases, such as ulcerative colitis and rheumatoid arthritis. The specific nomenclature of the four humors and their underlying assumptions are not medically valid, but the thematic idea of balance and restoration of normal regulatory function is well preserved.

[33] Hildegard and Matthew Fox, *Hildegard of Bingen's Book of Divine Works with Letters and Songs* (Santa Fe, NM: Bear & Co., 1987).

[34] Hildegard of Bingen, Book of Divine Works 4, 21 quoted in Fiona Bowie, Oliver Davies, and Hildegard, *Hildegard of Bingen: An Anthology* (London: SPCK, 1990), 29.

[35] Hildegard of Bingen, *Scivias, III, 6, 33*, quoted in ibid., 32.

Word manifests itself in every creature."[36] This power flowing through all living things connects the material and spiritual realms. Coursing through the body is the healing, greening power of God.

Sweet discovered an odd resonance between the outlook of this medieval saint and the world of her Laguna Honda patients, a complementarity between the "fast medicine" of her medical school training and the "slow medicine" she learned from Hildegard. In fact, she realized that the hospital was itself a physical legacy of Hildegard's medicine. Laguna Honda had once been San Francisco's almshouse. It had been built much as a medieval monastery/infirmary might have been. It had a central chapel, large open wards for the patients, and grounds for ambulatory patients to wander or work in. It included the elements of a village or a community, with a garden, orchards, greenhouse, aviary, and barnyard with resident animals. It retained a structure that suggested the residents were guests. The ramshackle premises offered a spectrum of activities that seemed decidedly non-medical in character.

Patients of last resort—those too poor to pay their way or those for whom modern medicine had already done its best—fetched up in this vestigial remnant of Hildegard's world. They came to be warehoused or die or, as Sweet discovered, sometimes to flourish. She reports on patients whose health was renewed by peeling away accretions of medication, reading carefully over their thick and often contradictory medical records, attending to their diet, listening to personal and spiritual aspirations, fostering human connections.

None of us want to forego fast medicine for the things it is so astoundingly good at. When we are blinded by cataracts, invaded by bacterial infection, struck down with a heart attack or in need of a new joint, we are fortunate not to live even one century earlier, so long as we are fortunate also to have the insurance policy and economic location that fast medicine often requires. When the problem is managing diabetes, back pain, the effects of chemotherapy, or virtually any condition to which doctors have chosen to attach the prefix "chronic," the case is quite different. Going on hospital rounds in an acute care ward, one may watch an impressive medical team grappling with patients almost all of whom, underlying their insurance-constrained few day stay for a fast medicine fix, suffered from slow medicine

---

[36]Gabriele Uhlein and Hildegard, *Meditations with Hildegard of Bingen*, New Age Mystics (Santa Fe, NM: Bear & Co., 1982), 49.

afflictions: addiction, uncontrolled glucose levels, constant pain, depression, a long list of conditions that are "refractive." That is, they are not going away under any treatment on order here. Faith, friendship, community, and care rarely cure the things that kill us quickly. They are sovereign medicine for what kills us slowly.

Such was Hildegard's counsel. What Laguna Honda gave Sweet was the gift of time with her patients. Hildegard taught her to use the time not only to look for new treatments to add, but to consider what was blocking the path of *viriditas* and how to free it. This might mean dropping a medication whose rationale was unclear, finding a more comfortable mattress to improve each night's sleep, replacing shoes that made walking painful, fostering work in the open air. It might mean going back to a medical fork in the path where a misguided treatment had become the source of its own illness.

Viriditas is not a medical term. It exists on another plane. But it dovetails suggestively with some contemporary medical insights. For instance, until relatively recently it was assumed that strokes—in which bleeding in the brain damages regions responsible for motion or activity (typically on one side of the body)—inflicted permanent damage, because the injured portions of the brain were exclusively responsible for the lost capacities. Rehabilitation might bring some limited recovery, but the die had largely been cast.

Edward Taub discovered that the then current scientific consensus behind this view was incorrect.[37] The brain has a previously unsuspected neuroplasticity that in many cases allows much more dramatic recovery from strokes. Such recovery is dependent on what he called "constraint induced" movement. That is, the affected limb has to be relentlessly and repetitively moved to essentially reactivate neurological patterns that control its activity. Those patterns, the brain "wiring" that controls an arm, say, may by such practice be built up in a different part of the brain than they were originally located. Or they may be reinstated in their original location, where the cells had not been irretrievably damaged, but only stunned into quiescence for a while. After a stroke, an arm may be unresponsive when the patient tries to move it, and so the patient gets used to not using it. This "learned disuse" is the downside of neurological plasticity, for the connections in the still-viable nerve cells atrophy and are effectively lost. That wiring has

---

[37]See Chapter Five, "Midnight Resurrections: Stroke Victims Learn to Move and Speak Again," in *The Brain That Changes Itself: Stories of Personal Triumph from the Frontiers of Brain Science*, ed. Norman Doidge (New York: Viking, 2007).

to be reawakened, or inscribed in a new location. This amazing plasticity looks a lot like a kind of *viriditas*: a self-healing dynamic in which the brain re-wires itself, a dynamic that requires trust and hope to activate.

Our immune systems are impressive forms of *viriditas*: self-healing, self-cleansing networks that fight off disruption and foster restorative growth. We have a growing list of autoimmune diseases, cases where our immune systems have been triggered for often mysterious reasons to target our own healthy cells and organs. These represent a branch of medicine that recalls Hildegard's idea of health and sickness as keyed not to noxious invaders but to the proper balance in our natural processes.

Sweet tells the story of Terry, who had lived on the streets of San Francisco, struggled with addiction, and was caught up in an abusive relationship. After twenty-eight visits to the emergency room in one year, Terry landed in Laguna Honda hospital with a deep ulcer across her back. Sweet said "It was so deep that at the bottom of it I could see bone, Terry's spine. It was filled with all this decayed tissue from her failed skin grafts. It was really too big to treat. It would have to heal on its own. I had nothing left in my little black bag." She remembered thinking "this sore is a catastrophe, and it is probably the end of Terry."[38]

But then she thought about *viriditas* and this idea that coursing through Terry's body was an invisible power of life and healing.[39] She thought Hildegard would just remove what was in the way of *viriditas*: fear, uncertainty hopelessness, medications she did not absolutely need, the pressure on the wound from lying on her back (removed by lying on a prone gurney). She would fortify the basics: good nutrition and plenty of rest. That was the prescription she applied. The resultant healing appeared magical to Sweet: slow, steady, comprehensive. "It took a long time. It took two and a half years. But Terry was not in a hurry, and neither were we."[40] At the end of that time, Terry reunited with her family and never returned to the streets.

Sweet noted that premodern medicine took it as a rule of thumb that an illness took as long to heal as it had taken to develop.[41] Depending on how Terry's sickness was defined, as a bed sore, a poor self-image or "what I really

---

[38] The preceding quotes and this one are from Victoria Sweet, "The Efficiency of Inefficiency," https://www.youtube.com/watch?v=VA08kzp7tSg.
[39] This paragraph paraphrased from Victoria Sweet, *God's Hotel: A Doctor, a Hospital, and a Pilgrimage to the Heart of Medicine* (New York: Riverhead Books, 2012), 106–7.
[40] Sweet, "The Efficiency of Inefficiency."
[41] Sweet, *God's Hotel: A Doctor, a Hospital, and a Pilgrimage to the Heart of Medicine*, 109.

believe it was—as some deep spiritual wound, two and a half years was just about right."[42] The dramatic against all odds healing of her back depended on another healing process that had taken place alongside it.[43] This was a change in temperament or spirit that grew as Terry put alcohol, drugs, and her abusive relationship behind her. Her physical change depended on a transformation that was making her whole and even happy, in a more encompassing way, even while she was still bedridden. Ever after, Sweet says, "instead of focusing on my patient vaguely surrounded by his environment ... I stepped back and focused on the environment surrounding my patient."[44] Fast medicine and slow medicine could work together in the same way our vision coordinates the input of two eyes, to produce a deeper field of vision, and a better form of health care.[45]

References

Ackerknecht, Erwin Heinz. *A Short History of Medicine.* Revised and expanded ed. Baltimore, MD: Johns Hopkins University Press, 2016.

Ackerknecht, Erwin Heinz. *Medicine at the Paris Hospital, 1794-1848.* Baltimore, MD: Johns Hopkins Press, 1967.

Berger, Margret, and Hildegard. *Hildegard of Bingen: On Natural Philosophy and Medicine: Selections from Cause Et Cure.* Library of Medieval Women. Cambridge; Rochester, NY: D.S. Brewer, 1999.

Blevins, Steve M., and Michael S. Bronze. "Robert Koch and the 'Golden Age' of Bacteriology." [In English U6—ctx_ver=Z39.88-2004&ctx_enc=info%3Aofi%2Fenc%3AUTF-8&rfr_id=info%3Asid%2Fsummon.serialssolutions.com&rft_val_fmt=info%3Aofi%2Ffmt%3Akev%3Amtx%3Ajournal&rft.genre=article&rft.atitle=Robert+Koch+and+the+%E2%80%98golden+age%E2%80%99+of+bacteriology&rft.jtitle=International+journal+of+infectious+diseases&rft.au=Blevins%2C+Steve+M&rft.au=Bronze%2C+Michael+S&rft.date=2010-09-01&rft.issn=1201-9712&rft.volume=14&rft.issue=9&rft.spage=e744&rft.epage=e751&rft_id=info:doi/10.1016%2Fj.ijid.2009.12.003&rft.externalDBID=ECK1-s2.0-S1201971210023143&rft.externalDocID=1_s2_0_S1201971210023143&paramdict=en-us U7—Journal

---

[42]Ibid.
[43]Material in this paragraph is paraphrased from ibid., 113.
[44]Ibid., 112.
[45]Sweet, "The Efficiency of Inefficiency."

Article]. *International journal of infectious diseases* 14, no. 9 (2010): e744–e51.

Bowie, Fiona, Oliver Davies, and Hildegard. *Hildegard of Bingen: An Anthology*. London: SPCK, 1990.

Curnow, Trevor. "The Cult of Asclepius: Its Origins and Early Development." [In English]. *Bulletin of the John Rylands Library (2014)* 89 (2013): 67–83.

Doidge, Norman. *The Brain That Changes Itself: Stories of Personal Triumph from the Frontiers of Brain Science*. New York: Viking, 2007.

Draper, John William. *History of the Conflict between Religion and Science*. 5th ed. New York: D. Appleton and Company, 1875.

Duval, John F., Lawrence M. Opas, Thomas J. Nasca, Paul Foster Johnson, and Kevin B. Weiss. "Report of the Si2025 Task Force." *Journal of Graduate Medical Education* 9, no. 6s (2017): 11–57.

Flanagan, Sabina. *Hildegard of Bingen, 1088-1179: A Visionary Life*. 2nd ed. London; New York: Routledge, 1998.

Harrison, Peter. *The Bible, Protestantism, and the Rise of Natural Science*. Cambridge; New York: Cambridge University Press, 1998.

Hayum, Andrée. *The Isenheim Altarpiece: God's Medicine and the Painter's Vision*. Princeton Essays on the Arts. Princeton, NJ: Princeton University Press, 1989.

Hildegard, and Matthew Fox. *Hildegard of Bingen's Book of Divine Works with Letters and Songs*. Santa Fe, NM: Bear & Co., 1987.

King, Stephen. *Trust the Process: A History of Clinical Pastoral Education as Theological Education* Lanham, MD: University Press of America 2007.

Lewis, C.S. *The Discarded Image: An Introduction to Medieval and Renaissance Literature*. Cambridge: Cambridge University Press, 1967.

Ludmerer, Kenneth M. "Abraham Flexner and Medical Education." [In English]. *Perspectives in Biology and Medicine* 54, no. 1 (2011): 8–16.

Morris, G. Scott, and Jim Wallis. *Care: How People of Faith Can Respond to Our Broken Health System*. Grand Rapids, MI: Eerdmans, William B. Publishing Company, 2022.

Newbigin, Lesslie. *Foolishness to the Greeks: The Gospel and Western Culture*. Wcc Mission Series; No. 6. Geneva: World Council of Churches, 1986.

Oren, Ohad, Bernard J. Gersh, and Deepak L. Bhatt. "On the Pearls and Perils of Sub-Subspecialization." *The American Journal of Medicine* 133, no. 2 (2020): 158–9.

Peterson, Derrick. "Galileo Again: Reevaluating Galileo's Conflict with the Church and Its Significance for Today." *Cultural Encounters: A Journal of Theology and Culture* 13, no. 1 (2017): 25–47.

Riddle, John M. "Theory and Practice in Medieval Medicine." In *Viator Medieval and Renaissance Studies: Volume 5 (1974)*, 161–88. Berkeley: University of California Press, 2023.

Risse, Guenter B. *Mending Bodies, Saving Souls: A History of Hospitals*. New York: Oxford University Press, 1999.

Schubert, Michael. *The Isenheim Altarpiece: History—Interpretation—Background*. English ed. Hudson Stuttgart: SteinerBooks; SchneiderEditionen, 2017. doi:9781621482093.

Science, The American Academy for the Advancement of. "Science and Religion: The Draper-White Conflict Thesis." https://youtu.be/ZLoZc5DIU9o.

Sullivan, Lawrence Eugene. *Healing and Restoring : Health and Medicine in the World's Religious Traditions*. New York London: Macmillan; Collier Macmillan, 1989.

Sweet, Victoria. *God's Hotel: A Doctor, a Hospital, and a Pilgrimage to the Heart of Medicine*. New York: Riverhead Books, 2012.

Sweet, Victoria. *Rooted in the Earth, Rooted in the Sky: Hildegard of Bingen and Premodern Medicine*. Studies in Medieval History and Culture. New York: Routledge, 2006.

Sweet, Victoria. "The Efficiency of Inefficiency." https://www.youtube.com/watch?v=VA08kzp7tSg.

Swing, Susan R., Stephen G. Clyman, Eric S. Holmboe, and Reed G. Williams. "Advancing Resident Assessment in Graduate Medical Education." [In English]. *Journal of Graduate Medical Education* 1, no. 2 (2009): 278–86.

Thomas, Lewis. *The Youngest Science: Notes of a Medicine-Watcher*. Oxford; New York: Oxford University Press, 1985.

Uhlein, Gabriele, and Hildegard. *Meditations with Hildegard of Bingen*. New Age Mystics. Santa Fe, NM: Bear & Co., 1982.

White, Andrew Dickson. *A History of the Warfare of Science with Theology in Christendom*. 2 vols. New York; London: D. Appleton and company, 1932.

4

Pain, Prayer, and Placebo

Chapter Outline

Where Does It Hurt? Distinguishing Pain and Suffering	68
Placebo and Prayer	73
The Therapy of Other Agency	76
What Kind of Prayer?	80
Full Spectrum Healing	82
Beyond Medicine	84

When your back hurts constantly, you make an appointment to see a doctor. When your heart aches with anxiety or grief, you may reach out to a counselor or a pastor. It is not always easy to segregate pain for our bodies and existential suffering for our spirits. Our friend, Gary Strichartz, has a unique perspective on these topics.[1] A professor of anesthesia, his lab at Harvard Medical School studied cellular mechanisms essential to the instigation and persistence of pain. Later in his career, he attended seminary, in order to be ordained in the Unitarian Universalist community and to serve as a chaplain in the same hospital system where his research was based. As he explains it, he has two lanyards with two different name tags. One labels him as a physician/researcher, the other as a religious chaplain. He has become a full spectrum healer, because the suffering he studied overflowed the disciplinary

---

[1] We regularly invite Dr. Strichartz to speak in our class, occasions when we always learn along with the students. He became a student and friend of Mark's when he attended Andover Newton Theological School. In the next section of this chapter, "Where Does It Hurt?," we draw freely on insights into the physiology of pain that we have gained from Dr. Strichartz.

boundaries we place on it. His research and pastoral experience converge in the same conviction: there is no mind-body dualism, no clear segregation of physiological pain and spiritual suffering.

Where Does It Hurt? Distinguishing Pain and Suffering

Even though physical pain and existential suffering are often divided by profession, they exist together in lived experience. Medical and religious terminology, which otherwise can diverge so much, intermingle here. Where pain is chronic, debilitating, or where the medical prognosis is discouraging and even terminal, medical vocabulary widens its horizon. It begins to be sprinkled with terms like quality of life, despair, hope, and meaning. Religious talk of deliverance and salvation, which is often evoked for moral, existential, or eschatological questions, turns poignantly concrete in face of an individual's bodily distress. How can God heal *this*, this tumor, this arthritis, this wound?

Pain and suffering are not the same thing. They are sadly cumulative, and one can be added to the other. The person struggling with purposelessness, experiencing the loss of a loved one, processing an adverse prognosis, or feeling profound guilt may feel deep distress but enjoy perfect outward health, with no twinge of physical discomfort. Yet they are in anguish at every instant. They are suffering. Suffering may be caused by physical pain and it can exacerbate or even instigate physical pain, but it is located in a cognitive-emotional and spiritual space. Suffering has always been a tributary source of religious thought and practice. As an inescapable, universal reality, it prompts reflection on whether any remedy exists, not to bring temporary respite, but as a definitive ultimate solution.

In our age, pain and its treatment have devolved more into the medical realm and existential suffering and its relief more into the religious one. Mental health, with its internal poles of "talk therapy" (cognitive-behavioral therapy) and drug treatments, forms a kind of middle ground between them.[2] For those who wish to keep religion and medicine entirely separate,

---

[2] See a sensitive treatment of these two sides of psychiatry in T. M. Luhrmann, *Of Two Minds: An Anthropologist Looks at American Psychiatry*, 1st Vintage Books ed. (New York: Vintage Books,

bodily pain and suffering are the province of medicine and the province of religion is to offer whatever solace may be found in face of all that medicine cannot treat, particularly suffering that is not physiological in origin (guilt, despair, meaninglessness).

Pain itself comes in different forms. At base, pain is a lifeline, a kind of guardian angel that sends a life-saving signal of danger to the body. It tells us that the coffee is too hot, that the steak knife has sliced into a finger, and that the morning's yardwork necessitates some ibuprofen. In the medical world, pain figures primarily in this alert mode. We discuss our pains with our doctors to help diagnose a possible threat to our life or health. The pain communicates and doctor and patient interpret what it is saying. We want to know if it is sending a transient, nagging message of indigestion or setting off a fire alarm for a heart attack. Sometimes, where the source of the pain is unclear, the pain itself must not be entirely relieved. Doctors need the channel of communication open for diagnosis, or analgesics might be dangerous for conditions that have not been ruled out.

Pain may even come to have emotionally positive significance. An extreme marathoner, a woman in childbirth, and someone undertaking a taxing medical rehabilitation regimen that promises restoration: the acute discomfort these persons experience is suffused with meaning and integral to good effects. So distinct are pain and suffering that the organic injury that can be the source of pain or disability may reside entirely in one person and the attendant suffering predominantly in another. People in coma states after traumatic injury are not actively aware of physiological pain in their bodies, but their loved ones sharply experience grief and anxiety—often with physical manifestations.

This holistic perspective is expressed in our physiology itself. Pain is not simply an inexorable response to an insult to our bodies from outside. Our experience of pain is the result of a two-way interaction. Nonnegotiable sensations travel "up" our neurological system, but their character may be dampened or amplified by responses that travel "down" that same system.[3] Tissue damage registers in nerve receptors in our body (our skin, for instance), that then transmit this stimulus up our spinal cord to various

---

2001).
[3] For a general description of this physiology, see Howard L. Fields, "Setting the Stage for Pain: Allegorical Tales from Neuroscience," in *Pain and Its Transformations: The Interface of Biology and Culture*, ed. Sarah Coakley and Kay Kaufman Shelemay (Cambridge, MA: Harvard University Press, 2007).

locations in our brains. Such input itself comes via two classes of nociceptors: a "fast" variety, that communicates location and intensity and prompts reflexive action, and a "slow" variety that connects to portions of the brain more related to emotions and learning. We can observe both of these by using a fingernail from one hand to sharply pinch the web of skin between thumb and index finger on the other hand. The initial sharp pain will be followed by a lingering dull ache. While sensations rise from our bodily periphery to be registered in our brains, messages also flow downward from the brain through various mechanisms that either inhibit the continued transmission of the pain stimulation signals or enhance their intensity. That descending modulation works primarily through the application or blocking of substances that attach to receptors that would otherwise be transmitting the pain sensations.

Pain stimulates areas of the brain producing changes in heart rate and blood pressure, and also affecting the production of emotions, notably fear and anxiety. These effects, which are a major part of the pain experience, are themselves subject to counterstimulations that reduce (or amplify) those aspects of the experience. This pain modulatory system assures that the same bodily events do not necessarily equate to the same pain, even in the same person. If you repeat the pinching experiment, and then immediately gently rub the knuckles near the pinched skin, you will notice the lingering pain diminishes more rapidly. The rubbing sets up competing neurological messages that modify the experienced sensation of pain, a medical intervention familiar to parents who intuitively rub where their child receives a bump. "Kissing where it hurts" is sound neurological advice, as one simultaneous sensation can modify the experience of another.

The existence of such a two-way modulation process helps to explain why people experience pain dramatically differently. A wide variety of factors can affect the function of this modulation, from genetic dispositions, to social-cultural contexts, to quality of sleep, to physiological disease processes, and pre-existing psychological conditions. Most particularly, major trauma and repetitive injury can sensitize or reset this modulatory system itself, so that sensory input that would not register as pain or as debilitating pain in most people (or in the same person prior to their sensitization) now causes severe pain. In this respect there is a learned or conditioned aspect to pain. The "tuning" of our pain modulation systems may be affected by non-genetic inheritance of traumatic effects across generations—a form of epigenetics.[4] The experienced effects of physical injury and trauma can be intensified when caused by or associated with injustice or indifference from those around us. The physical pain experienced by an abused child has a different character from the same biological injury suffered in an accident or from disease.

Pain becomes pathological when its presence and effects constitute the primary problem that needs healing. Rather than indicating an issue, pain itself becomes the wound. Like the endless piercing noise of a smoke alarm in the absence of a fire, it crowds out other thought or action. In autoimmune diseases, the defense mechanism against bacterial or viral threats has turned against healthy tissues. Chronic or debilitating pain is a kind of autoimmune reaction. Our protector has become an enemy. Phantom limb pain is a dramatic illustration of this phenomenon, with the pain sensed as originating in and being felt through a limb that is entirely absent. Pain occurs with no "objective" input. The perceived pain is being produced by the system that responds to it.

Though the ascending and descending pain pathways link our bodies and brains with each other and mediate our relation with the surrounding environment, all pain is "in our heads." It is in our brains that pain is perceived and its meaning for us expressed. When addressing pathological pain, the discourse of the medical world migrates again toward the religious one. Pain is an experience that is more than a sensation. The concrete perception of the input received by our brains will depend on a range of factors, some biological and some more associated with context, values, and culture. It is not surprising that religious faith and practices loom large among those factors.

How then do religion and medicine interact in the healing of pain and suffering? From the start, it is important to acknowledge that their interaction is not always synergistic, above all because their ultimate ends are not identical. Sometimes their goals may not be directly related or they may even pull in opposite directions. Health is the *telos* of medicine, but virtually all forms of religious devotion place some goods above bodily health. Religious faithfulness sometimes commends behavior that results in pain or suffering in adherents. This may involve forms of asceticism for self-formation or

---

[4] The most familiar articulation of this is found in Bessel A. Van der Kolk, *The Body Keeps the Score: Brain, Mind, and Body in the Healing of Trauma* (New York: Viking, 2014).

actions that place one's love for neighbors and God above one's own physical health and emotional peace. What counts as spiritual well-being can run counter to physical flourishing. Most people place some things above optimal health and length of life. We may all do this unthinkingly, in falling into poor nutrition choices or in avoiding exercise. But people may do this with considered purpose, choosing a shorter but more conscious path to death in a final illness, or in persisting in significant activities or work that may negatively affect health.

Theologian Stanley Hauerwas suggests that the true measure of well-being for Christians is their capacity to participate in community with others and in communion with God.[5] That those who are healthy in a community care for those that are not, and that those who are ill (for whom isolation itself is often a major co-morbidity) retain interest in and connection with the wider world—these are part of the core definition of "health" for the Christian community itself, as well as for each of its members. Accordingly, the person whose medical condition is dire, but retains the capacity for prayer, care, and community, is healthier in one significant measure compared to those estranged from God and others, not at peace with themselves, even if physiologically robust. At the extreme, one seeks healing of the first type over that of the second. It is religiously meaningful to speak of wellness *in* suffering.

By contrast, strictly medical aims can disregard or subordinate religious ones. Medical healing can proceed effectively with no need for religious reference, or in face of religious resistance. The appendectomy, conducted with complete indifference to spirituality on the part of both surgeon and patient, reliably preserves health and well-being. The blood donation administered over religious objections prevents death.

Most of the time, we argue, religious commitment undergirds health, and medical care is more effective when it recognizes the spiritual dimension. There is a natural consonance here. Unnecessary conflict between religion and medicine is itself a negative factor that adds to the sum of human pain and suffering, as their cooperation subtracts from it.

---

[5] Stanley Hauerwas, "Suffering Presence: Twenty-Five Years Later," in *Healing to All Their Flesh*, ed. Jeff Levin and Keith Meador (Conshohocken, PA: Templeton Press, 2013).

Placebo and Prayer

Much discussion of medicine and theology has focused on the category of the miraculous, the sudden reversal of disease or injury following an appeal to divine aid, a cure unexpected and inexplicable in medical terms. Throughout the history of medicine in the Christian world, medical treatments and divine healing were generally affirmed as both part of a common standard of care. In the development of hospitals, for instance, treatments (according to the medicine of the time) and spiritual support went hand in hand and were rarely opposed to each other.[6] Miracles were part of this landscape, marking a difference in degree of divine healing, but not a difference in kind from less dramatic cases of "normal" medicine where the divine was also believed to have a hand.

In the modern period, skepticism about divine action pitted faith and medicine against each other, in the sense that divine action could be credited as a real factor only in the extreme case where medical causality itself could be effectively ruled out. Certification of miracles in the Roman Catholic Church—in the investigation of claims for sainthood or documentation at a pilgrimage center like Lourdes, for instance—came to involve extensive medical documentation. The documentation was meant to provide proof for the absence of a plausible medical explanation.[7] Such emphasis on the extraordinary, on miracles as a theological "proof of concept," could lead both medicine and theology to pay less attention to everyday realities, where the inputs and outputs may not be so definitively distinguished. That emphasis implies the relevance of the spiritual is rare and exceptional, when we are arguing it is consistent and normal.

Theologically, we affirm the reality of divine action that goes beyond our understanding. But theology is even more profoundly concerned with articulating God's love and support for human well-being as a universal feature, not an extraordinary and episodic one. For miracle to be the only mode of divinely aided healing would reflect a great constraint on God's power (limiting its exercise to rare occasions) and a limitation on the scope of God's love (suggesting that it extends only to a few). One may believe

---

[6] As we argued in Chapter 3.
[7] For an interesting review, including a discussion of the criteria for "cure," see B. François, E.M. Sternberg, and E. Fee, "The Lourdes Medical Cures Revisited," *Journal of the History of Medicine and Allied Sciences* 69, no. 1 (2014): 135–62.

miracles are real and yet regard them as exemplary, rather than exhaustive of divine concern for healing. This belief in a consistent and universal exercise of divine influence points toward an interest in the statistically more "normal" forms of spiritual support for healing. On the medical side, meanwhile, there is obviously primary interest in religious activities whose impact on health might be consistent and measurable, and so possibly integrated into an evidence-based clinical practice. We turn now to two topics that provide an illuminating perspective on just these issues of consistency and replicability, rather than the extreme and exceptional. These are aspects of the medical and religious worlds that are so ubiquitous as to be almost invisible: placebo and prayer.

Prayer is the most widely practiced—and perhaps most widely prescribed—religious "treatment" for illness. It is an enormous cumulative input to the bio-medical reality. Even those for whom prayer is not a regular feature of their lives often practice it in the face of illness or medical crisis. Such widespread prayer and God's supposed sensitivity to it correspond to the theological expectation that there should be some such widespread divine activity on behalf of the afflicted. However, from a medical and scientific perspective, this enormous volume of spiritual activity explicitly directed toward healing lacks any clearly measurable effect, the kind of evidence medicine depends on.[8]

The placebo phenomenon is a long-recognized and increasingly researched effect, with reference to virtually all medical contexts, from clinical trials of drugs to bed-side practice.[9] Placebos are popularly understood to be sham medical treatments, a sugar pill or the injection of an inactive substance given to unknowing patients to mimic an actual therapy. Placebos' role in medical trials originated in a belief that the placebo group functioned as a control group, for whom nothing of medical relevance was being done. It long ago became evident that placebos do not equate with doing nothing, for they can be accompanied by objective changes in recipients. Three-armed experimental trials (in which one group receives no treatment whatsoever, another receives a placebo, and a third receives the target treatment) regularly demonstrate that placebos produce an improvement over that found in the absence of any treatment at all. Therapies

---

[8]In this connection, see the discussion of randomized controlled trials of prayer's effect in Chapter 6.
[9]Daniel E. Moerman, *Meaning, Medicine, and the "Placebo Effect"*, Cambridge Studies in Medical Anthropology (Cambridge; New York: Cambridge University Press, 2002).

that are subject to such controlled evaluation need to demonstrate not just that their benefit exceeds that of doing nothing, but that it exceeds the benefit of the *appearance* of a treatment, the placebo.

That those treated with a "fake" agent may show marked improvements over those who received no treatment at all, even similar benefits to those who received actual medications, is one of the more consistently replicated results in medical literature.[10] This measurable and ubiquitous effect notoriously lacks any agreed causal explanation. For this reason, its reality is disputed or, often, tacitly ignored. Yet most physicians acknowledge that they have incorporated it at some time as an element in their clinical practice.[11] Part of the challenge for research into the placebo effect is that what is being studied is an unavoidable active ingredient in every explicit medical intervention, responsible for some variable fraction of the benefit produced by any of them. Patients are always responding not just to the molecular composition of a drug or the physical effects of a surgery, but to their belief that they have received an effective treatment.

Some pre-modern medical treatments have been found to have scientifically intelligible mechanisms of action that account for real effects. However, those without any such mechanism, still had the hardly negligible power of the placebo effect.

Serious research on placebos continues to grow, as do attempts to harness them as treatment modalities.[12] This interest perhaps is related to an increasing openness within the medical world to non-sectarian spiritual input, and "alternative medicine" more broadly. But some medical professionals deny the reality of the placebo phenomenon, contending that it is a kind of optical illusion, a statistical reflection of the fact that many ills, especially those that are self-reported, simply get better over time.[13] Indeed, the placebo phenomenon is not equally evident across all medical conditions. Placebo effects for the healing of a ruptured appendix, leukemia, or a massive

---

[10] The changes are typically positive, but a "nocebo" effect of negative responses is also observed—including, for instance patients experiencing the side effects of the medicine they (falsely) believe they are taking. Luana Colloca and Arthur J. Barsky, "Placebo and Nocebo Effects," *The New England Journal of Medicine* 382, no. 6 (2020): 554–61.

[11] See for instance A. Raz, E. Raikhel, and R.D. Anbar, "Placebos in Medicine: Knowledge, Beliefs, and Patterns of Use," *McGill Journal of Medicine* 11, no. 2 (2008): 206–11.

[12] It is not surprising that a great many placebo studies deal with pain, since this is a condition endemic across many different medical conditions and one where ethical frameworks are clearer (subjects agree to participate knowing that they may or may not receive a placebo).

[13] Perhaps the best-known argument of this type is A. Hróbjartsson and P.C. Gøtzsche, "Is the Placebo Powerless?" *New England Journal of Medicine* 344, no. 21 (2001): 1594–602.

heart attack may exist. But there is little evidence for them, not least because it would be unethical to experimentally give placebos in place of proven treatments in life-threatening contexts. Yet even should one go so far as to suppose placebo effects are limited to conditions in large part defined by the patient's self-reported experience (levels of pain, ability to perform specific activities, quality of life), this would mean they apply to a large portions of medical conditions, including many of the most serious and chronic ones.[14]

Critics argue that placebo effects register only subjective self-reporting, that patients are experiencing no objective change in their physiological conditions and simply convince themselves to report their condition more positively. This seems implausible, since placebo effects are found in changed physiological measurements related to "hard core" objective conditions including high blood pressure, ulcers, and coronary artery disease. This includes placebo effects for "sham" surgeries.[15] Placebos, or peoples' reaction to them, can be shown to produce measurable physical changes in the *mechanisms* that account for their effect on symptoms.[16] For instance, patients whose pain was reduced on receipt of a placebo were found to have natural endorphins blocking pain receptors: the placebo produced the reduction in pain through the same physiological mechanism that a drug produces. Administering naloxone, which blocks endorphins from such receptors, reversed the effect of the placebo, just as it would a chemical opiate. The placebo response does not just change cognitive perspective: it changes and moves molecules in the body.

The Therapy of Other Agency

Placebo and prayer are tantalizing mirror images of each other. Where prayer's massive input has no easily measured empirical effect, the placebo's pervasively detected effect has no clear corresponding cause. Contemplating this picture, one of our students responded this way: "The placebo effect is a check drawn on the countless prayers offered each day for the sick, collectively and individually. It is a consistent, invisible divine thumb on

---

[14]See the discussion of "fast medicine" and "slow medicine" in Chapter 3.
[15]On blood pressure, ulcers, coronary artery disease, and surgeries, see Chapters 5 and 6 in Moerman, *Meaning, Medicine, and the "Placebo Effect"*.
[16]For information in the balance of this paragraph, see ibid., 105–7.

the scales of health." Miracles are decisive and happen only to the few. The placebo effect is significant, if rarely determinative, and manifests for almost all. The startled student's linking of placebo with prayer stimulated us to explore the connections further, and the direct interface of religious practice and medicine.

We can begin with our discussion of pain earlier in this chapter. We saw there that there is a significant dimension of physiological self-modulation in response to injury or disease. Our bodies can mobilize natural opiates to temper pain, just as they mobilize other healing responses in our immune system or in anti-inflammatory processes. We saw that many factors could influence that process, including emotional, cognitive, and social ones. This plasticity offers a direct window for religious practice to interface with the physiological process. Spiritual and religious orientations may enhance such healing self-modulations (or, in some forms, inhibit them). That is, there is a spiritual "immune response" to bodily trauma.

The spiritual immune response operates across a range of more and less explicitly religious practices, as it also ranges from a narrow focus on the single body as a self-contained system to a perspective that stresses wider integration. Specifically, in relation to pain, practices oriented to breath control and focused concentration (repetition of a mantra or a prayer) can modulate physiological responses and so modulate the severity of discomfort. One vein of prayer can be seen as self-medication of this sort, and could be interpreted as confined to the subjective recesses of the prayer/patient. Agent and beneficiary are one. That is, the benefits of prayer are found in those who pray (and can be seen as a subset of the health benefits of religious practice understood more widely). The medical benefits involved here have been quite extensively documented in the area of mind-body medicine.[17]

But what of prayer's relation to other agency? Prayer as part of a spiritual immune system is important. But it leaves aside the question, so important to many religious people, of relation with others and particularly with God. Can one's prayer be healing for another? The medical evidence for placebo takes us a step beyond prayer as self-regulation and toward this relational dimension. Placebos are generally an *external* treatment. Though the response to placebos takes effect within the patient, where the result is measured, the application is *external*. That is to say, this healing dynamic

---

[17]Herbert Benson and Marg Stark, *Timeless Healing: The Power and Biology of Belief* (New York: Scribner, 1996).

necessarily includes the intercession of other agents, and to this extent is more open to divine agency. Placebos are, by definition, *not* self-administered. They depend on the activity of supposed qualities in the treatments (the contents in the pill or the injection), and on the attitude of those who commend and apply them. Placebo effects turn on relationships. Whatever trust or expectation exists in the patient, conducive to healing, is produced by the action of others *in whom* the patient takes there to be healing authority.

Agency seems to be a central component of the placebo effect. Another person, whose relevant knowledge and skill I respect, and whose benevolent intention toward me I trust, has acted to heal me. I am an object of care to another. The pill, treatment, or practice is the medium through which that intention is carried out. In place of "placebo effect," one major placebo researcher prefers the term "meaning effect," with the suggestion that the patient is responding not to the supposed treatment, but to the meaning (as just described) surrounding it.[18] My relation with the agent and the agent's intention has transferred meaning to the substance I believe will realize that intention. Meaning is similarly what is essentially at issue when patients report greater benefit from a pill received under a brand name than from the same pill under a generic name. The meaning derives from a relational context. Placebo effects seem to depend upon a level of cognitive capacity. Alzheimer patients whose frontal cortex function has declined to a point that degrades cognitive function also experienced a decline in the placebo effect.[19] The healing benefits flow through our meaning-making capacities.

Both the other-directed aspect and the meaning element are illustrated in a study of pain relief after the extraction of wisdom teeth.[20] Patients were randomized to receive one of three substances: a placebo, an opiate antagonist (naloxone) that physiologically should make pain worse, or a narcotic pain reliever (fentanyl). The patients were told these were the three randomized options, and that the treatment they received might increase their pain, diminish it, or have no effect. The clinicians administering the injections and the questionnaires for patients to report their pain levels were (unbeknown to them) part of a further twist in the study.

---

[18] Phil Hutchinson and Daniel E. Moerman, "The Meaning Response, 'Placebo', and Methods," *Perspectives in Biology and Medicine* 61, no. 3 (2018): 361–78.
[19] A.J. Pardo-Cabello, V. Manzano-Gamero, and E. Puche-Canas, "Placebo: A Brief Updated Review," *Naunyn Schmiedeberg's Arch Pharmacol* 395, no. 11 (2022): 1343–56.
[20] R.H. Gracely, "Clinician's Expectations Influence Placebo Analgesia," *Lancet* 1, no. 8419 (1985): 43.

They were told that there was a shortage of fentanyl and so none of the first cohort of patients would be receiving actual fentanyl; for the later cohort of patients, all three options would be in play. Thus the dentists believed that in the first round no one would receive the opiate and in the second round patients *might* receive it. In truth, all patients were randomized to the three options.

The researchers compared the placebo response in the two groups of patients. Those who had received placebo injections from dentists certain they could not be receiving actual medication reported pain increasing dramatically from baseline. However, patients receiving the same placebo injections from clinicians who believed they might be receiving an analgesic reported a significant decrease in pain from the baseline level. In this case it appears to be the expectation (i.e., the awareness of a statistical possibility in the *clinician* that is the variable influencing the effect in the *patient*). For this purpose, it does not matter how or if patients were subliminally tipped off to the dentist's state of mind, only that it is the relation to the other and to the other's awareness or intent that is the operative factor.

When we view the placebo effect as a meaning response, it makes sense that there is not actually one placebo effect, but many. These can vary depending upon the cultural context. The German placebo effect in regard to ulcers is twice the world average and three times as high as in neighboring countries, but the German placebo effect in high blood pressure is among the lowest in the world.[21] This variation suggests that the meaning response, while operative in all people, can be effectively shaped by features like religious or cultural frameworks. The supposed division in which medicine deals with health and religion deals with meaning is not supportable: meaning is an inextricable element in healing and health.

With the evidence for the placebo as a meaning effect, there is nothing disparaging in considering spiritual and religious orientation under that same heading. One might even say that the meaning response is itself part of religious/worldview outlooks in the widest sense. The placebo response draws on a larger fund of meaning and assumptions, including those relating to doctors and medicine generally, as well as to specific doctors and specific treatments. Divine agency is both the most universally accessible and directly interested factor in this wider constellation of meaning. For the religious person, the conviction that this agent has specific care and healing intentions

---

[21] Moerman, *Meaning, Medicine, and the "Placebo Effect,"* 81–2.

for me is not something that must be established *de novo* in the context of illness. The attitude that one has toward God is a means by which God is able to foster healing in you. In the medical world, the placebo effect often registers as a kind of interference, noise that prevents a clearer determination of biological causation. But perhaps that effect simply reflects another dimension of causality—a mental and spiritual one—that is always at play. It is the unavoidable tip of a larger less visible iceberg.

What Kind of Prayer?

We have been arguing that religion, and specifically prayer, has a medically intelligible place in the healing process. Could we inquire further about whether some kinds of prayer have different effects than others? Some of the most interesting recent work in this area has been done by Marta Illueca. A pediatric gastroenterologist and an Episcopal priest, Illueca collaborated with one of us (Doolittle) to conduct a systematic review of prayer in the management of pain.[22] The review limited its scope to studies where prayer was defined as an active intervention on site (at the bedside) involving communication with a higher power and where pain was one of the specified outcome measures. The review categorized prayer according to four variables. These related to the source of the prayer material (scriptural or mantric), the target of the prayer (religious or secular), the mode or outlook of the prayer (active or passive), and the implementation form (receptive listening or personal expression).[23] One interesting finding of the review was that all prayer is not clinically equal. Some forms could be associated with differential levels of pain tolerance. For instance, passive forms of petitionary prayer ("take away the pain") did not decrease reported pain levels. Active forms ("help me to endure the pain") were, on the other hand, associated with higher pain tolerance than other forms of prayer or no prayer at all.[24]

In further work, Illueca has collaborated with a nonreligious clinical psychologist and pain researcher to develop and validate a scale to measure

---

[22] M. Illueca and B.R. Doolittle, "The Use of Prayer in the Management of Pain: A Systematic Review," *Journal of Religion and Health* 59, no. 2 (2020): 681–99.
[23] Ibid., 698.
[24] On active and passive prayer, see S.M. Meints et al., "An Experimental Investigation of the Relationships among Race, Prayer, and Pain," *Scandinavian Journal of Pain* 18, no. 3 (2018): 545–53.

pain-related prayer.[25] Unlike prior research, this scale distinguishes between active, passive, and neutral modes of prayer.[26] If research continues to confirm that active prayer is associated with significant pain relief together with improved coping, then the authors suggest scale-derived practical aids "could be used by chaplains and pastors to help individuals with chronic pain expand their prayer practices, including the adoption of an active style of prayer."[27] They have developed a "bedside prayer tool" that could be used by health care providers to "assist people in understanding their prayer style and how it relates to their pain experience."[28]

This research addresses religious interventions and their therapeutic potential for medical conditions (in this case pain). Illueca has also written about the other side of that coin: religious suffering that is unaddressed in medical treatment.[29] She explores the realm of spiritual affliction that she argues deserves medical recognition because it compromises human well-being, as well as negatively affecting other health outcomes. A sense of estrangement from God, alienation from spiritual peace, need for forgiveness, isolation from religious community or practice: these are conditions that entail real pain and suffering. But they often are beyond the border of consideration by health care providers.[30]

---

[25] S.M. Meints et al., "The Pain and Prayer Scale (Pprayers): Development and Validation of a Scale to Measure Pain-Related Prayer," *Pain Medicine* 24, no. 7 (2023): 862–71.
[26] The modes are active ("Help me to manage this pain"), passive ("Take my pain away"), and neutral ("May my body align with the universe's healing power").
[27] Meints et al., "The Pain and Prayer Scale (Pprayers): Development and Validation of a Scale to Measure Pain-Related Prayer," 869.
[28] Ibid. To see the tool, visit https://painandprayer.com/wp-content/uploads/2023/04/PainPrayerBrochureDraft8.pdf.
[29] M. Illueca, Y.S. Bradshaw, and D.B. Carr, "Spiritual Pain: A Symptom in Search of a Clinical Definition," *Journal of Religion and Health* 62, no. 3 (2023): 1920–32.
[30] One form of spiritual pain has been gaining some visibility in the medical world: moral injury. In addition to physical trauma and associated symptoms of anxiety and depression, many who experience those afflictions (or from having been witnesses or parties to others being so afflicted) suffer from a discrete additional trauma. This is a loss of meaning, a shattering of human connection, and a loss not only of a sense of safety, but of one's moral assumptions about one's self and the world. See Warren Kinghorn, "Combat Trauma and Moral Fragmentation: A Theological Account of Moral Injury," *Journal of the Society of Christian Ethics* 32, no. 2 (2012): 57–74; Larry Kent Graham, *Moral Injury: Restoring Wounded Souls* (Nashville: Abingdon Press, 2017).

Full Spectrum Healing

The landscape we have briefly sketched suggests some theological as well as medical reflections. As we noted earlier, placebo is a constant factor in virtually all medical interventions, to some degree tipping the scales toward a better clinical outcome. Prayer is a widespread human response to medical distress, for whose effectiveness it is hard to formulate evidence, short of the most extreme cases of miraculous healing. We suggest prayer and placebo should be seen as part of one continuous reality. To the theological question of why a God who is supposed to proactively care for all should offer healing aid only rarely and inexplicably, we could say that the placebo/meaning effect—responsive as it is to the belief in external beneficent intent—marks precisely that universally available support. It is granted indifferently, to the religious or nonreligious, if they open themselves to it, becoming more explicitly religious to the extent that it is sought from or associated with a divine agent.

We could put the same thing negatively, by reference to the famous example of Romanian orphanages where small children were provided with all the supposed essentials of life—food, clothing, shelter—but sickened and died at catastrophic rates because they were deprived of the "soft" features of care such as touch, eye contact, play.[31] Survival may be a biological imperative. But it appears that even the will to live, manifest throughout infant bodies in numberless paths of development, is sustained in us only by the example of others outside us signifying by their care and attention that they *desire* our health and our more than simply physical well-being. The placebo effect that is mediated not through the patient's assumptions, but through their care giver's mere expectation (the intravenous line *might* contain the fentanyl, when in fact it does not) begins to look *vicarious* in nature. Someone else's belief that I am receiving healing aid turns out to be healing for me even if not explicitly communicated to me.

A caregiver's belief that a treatment may help me is not clearly distinguishable on my part from a care giver's intention to help me, which motivates the treatment. Both have their own therapeutic power. This might help to explain Illueca's tentative findings that active prayer has more

---

[31]Charles A. Nelson, Nathan A. Fox, and Charles H. Zeanah, *Romania's Abandoned Children: Deprivation, Brain Development, and the Struggle for Recovery* (Cambridge, MA: Harvard University Press, 2014).

measured benefits in pain reduction than passive or neutral prayer: such prayer invites divine aid to assist the person and their care givers as they respond to the pain and so explicitly supports the expectation that such aid will come *through* the medical media as well as others. In addition to any other benefits, such prayer directly enlists divine beneficent intention "behind" existing treatment. Prayers for divine aid attach themselves concretely to whatever agents or substance might be taken to mediate that aid.

We saw that the placebo effect turns crucially on the caregiver's expressed or sensed attitude, but the patient's appropriation of this meaning is typically magnified by tangible agents that concretize it. This is the longstanding assumption in Christian practice, where tangible and sacramental signs (anointing with oil, reception of communion, laying on of hands) are acts of healing and associated with prayer. Believing that you are being prayed for or that God is benevolent toward you is one thing. Someone actively praying in your presence, or a community's ritual around you—these are ways of making that agency more tangible and available to your apprehension, both cognitively and implicitly.

The picture we have outlined is radically different from the common one that sees a baseline landscape of objective medical care, overlaid with a cloud of largely irrelevant (and certainly not evidence based) religious attitudes and practices that patients bring into play, and marked with occasional flashes of unexplained medical restorations that might be claimed as miracles. Instead, we see a spectrum of biological medical treatments, virtually every element of which already carries within it a smaller or larger dimension of "meaning effect" that enhances or limits its impact. That meaning effect scales up into more explicit religious or spiritual forms which are purposely aimed to focus (as a lens or a laser focuses) that meaning effect for healing. To speak of prayer as part of the placebo effect is not to denigrate it, but to validate it in terms accessible to medical understanding, without requiring religious people to take this description as exhaustive. Medical researchers have begun to turn from regarding placebo or meaning effects as complicating "static" in research toward considering them as treatment agents in their own right. To investigate the way that prayer might be tuned for its best medical effects is to follow in the same direction.

A religious patient or caregiver need not foreclose the hope of miracles. They can do so, however, in confidence that their absence does not mean that prayer is without effect. In truth, these prayers and the divine responsiveness they assume are active forces for healing, whose effect is seamlessly bound up with the medical treatments and other supports the afflicted person receives. Whether or not they decisively tip the balance between life and death, cure or loss—and miracle may be the extremely rare case where such a discrimination is even possible—spiritual supports are no less supports for healing than hydration.

Religious meaning is not limited to its effect on physical healing. Such meaning seamlessly "treats" forms of suffering and distress that go beyond biology and ultimately cannot be addressed by medicine. Insofar as spiritual means heal such spiritual afflictions, that primary treatment can have still further benefits for physical healing as a side effect. From this perspective, religious response to illness can consistently put a positive weight on the scales of physical healing, a difference that may or may not in any specific case be enough to shift the balance of the outcome. At the same time, that response addresses the needs that medicine itself cannot.

Beyond Medicine

Prayer and religious practice are directed to forms of healing that transcend illness and mortality, that go beyond them and can coexist with them. From a medical perspective the meaning effect may extend "up" into the realm of prayer. But from a religious perspective the reality of prayer, which is fundamentally devoted to spiritual peace and power, reconciliation with God and others, extends "down" from that sphere into the realm of physical healing as well. As God the creator stands behind the extraordinary biological processes of maintenance and repair in our bodies, so this God is implicated in the wider social-spiritual network of forces that extend the range of that healing, and enhance the effectiveness of medical interventions to repair or assist it.

The "alert" function of pain is a blessing of a healthy body. A neurological inability to feel pain is a serious disability, whose missing messages are a constant threat to safety. So, in a similar sense, religious visions of health see a positive role for certain kinds of distress. Remorse and concern over wrongdoing, commitment to ideals that lead us to be unhappy with the world as it is—these are forms of pain that are healthy and constructive, actively fostered in religious contexts. Indeed, we could say that learning to feel and care for other peoples' pain is an index of spiritual health, even though it may be a stress on one's own physical well-being. Pain becomes suffering when it lacks instrumental value (as in prompting me to move my fingers from the stove), and lacks integral meaning as part of a larger project (for instance required to achieve a worthy goal). Pain without meaning of these sorts becomes suffering, along with the spectrum of non-medical conditions of spiritual meaninglessness that lead bodily healthy people to despair.

In the same way that a body can suffer, so too can a community: a family, a church, a neighborhood. Communities "suffer" from the debilities and pain of members. The medical condition of those in a community affects its life, something economists recognize as lost productivity but which is a reality in all spheres. Features of the life of the community have their effects on individual members, as well as on the community as a whole. There is social suffering, whose pangs are felt most sharply by some parts of the community rather than others. As we look back at the Covid-19 pandemic, we are aware of the associated forms of loss it spread in our communities, and aware that these fell unevenly on their members. Medicine increasingly attends to this under the heading of social determinants of health, whether the determinant in question is access to health care itself, or increased liability to disease because of social location.

Christians take this reflection one step further and ask does God suffer? A God who cares for creation and who is intimately connected with it must, it seems, experience pain in a sense analogous to our "alert" pain. Such a God registers—not by distant inference, but by immediate awareness—what is unjust, wounding, and destructive for God's creatures. Human violence, hatred, and suffering are painful to God in that awareness sense, reflexively calling forth the exercise of the powers in the divine immune system against them. Christian belief affirms that God also participates in the meaningful pain borne in the service of restoration and healing. The incarnation, crucifixion, and resurrection are cardinal signs of this. In these respects, God suffers—experiences—redemptive pain. To love is to suffer. Every parent understands that. Anyone who has ever loved understands that. And such love is bound up in everything that gives our lives meaning.

But we have distinguished such experience from suffering in a deeper sense: pain with no viable "alert" function, debilitating pain that plays no constructive positive role, forms of spiritual despair or anguish that block participation in all of all life's goods. It would seem that this is one kind of suffering from which God would be exempt. The suffering born of despair or helplessness or ignorance is presumably a feature of our human finitude, a condition not shared by God.

This undeniable gap is a facet of faith. The theodicy question—how can a good God allow evil and suffering in the world?—can be posed as a logical issue. But it is basically an experiential one. It is a plaintive request that asks for the gap to be closed. "If God has a perspective in which the pains of the world are *not* suffering in that deeper sense, because taken up in wider significance, why won't God share it?" Christian theology has generally held that the full divine perspective can't be shared with humans, consistent with our capacities. But something equally extraordinary is possible: the human experience of unredeemed pain, its grief and loss, can be shared by God.

Nicholas Wolterstorff captures this view in his book *Lament for a Son*. Wolterstorff's twenty-five-year-old son died in a rock climbing accident in Austria. He writes about his son, but he could be writing about any other horrible tragedy:

> How is faith to endure, O God, when you allow all this scraping and tearing on us? You have allowed rivers of blood to flow, mountains of suffering to pile up, sobs to become humanity's song—all without lifting a finger that we could see . . . If you have not abandoned us, explain yourself.[32]

Later in the book, he attempts an answer. He writes,

> We strain to hear. But instead of hearing an answer, we catch sight of God himself scraped and torn. Through our tears, we see the tears of God.[33]

Christians believe that in Jesus, God enters into the world to experience it from the human side, including the elements of suffering that come from human limitation. God knows suffering not only through an empathetic awareness of what creatures experience (and such a sensation, on a universal level, is itself a divine capacity), but through participation in a unique human life subject to all its limitations. Paradoxical though it is, the word from the cross "My God, my God, why have you forsaken me?", indicates that in Jesus God has crossed the chasm of meaningless suffering to our side of it. Our problem is God's problem. This makes God's suffering not an intellectual abstraction, but a messy, irrevocable involvement in the narrative arc of history.

God does not exclusively have our human perspective, but God has become intrinsically bound to that perspective. So "the history of our world

---

[32]Nicholas Wolterstorff, *Lament for a Son* (Grand Rapids, MI: Wm B Eerdmans Publishing), 80.
[33]Ibid., 80.

is the history of our suffering together. Every act of evil extracts a tear from God, every plunge into anguish extracts a sob from God. But the history of our world is the history of our deliverance together. God's work to release himself from his suffering is his work to deliver the world from its agony; our struggle for joy and justice is our struggle to relieve God's sorrow." [34] This is a statement of faith. But the healing power of such faith can be empirically observed.

This chapter suggests that the religious impact on medical healing exists across a wide spectrum. It is broad and constant as a force mixed in with placebo or meaning effects as well as self-regulation in health care. Always including those effects, religious practice "scales up" to specific personal and community forms of prayer and ritual. These practices address forms of healing that go beyond the physical, including interpersonal and spiritual reconciliation. Healing of this sort has its own positive effects on medical well-being. Here the medical value derives from a non-medical one, coming precisely as the side effect of a resolution that takes place more on religious terms.

References

Benson, Herbert, and Marg Stark. *Timeless Healing: The Power and Biology of Belief*. New York: Scribner, 1996.

Colloca, Luana, and Arthur J. Barsky. "Placebo and Nocebo Effects." [In English]. *The New England Journal of Medicine* 382, no. 6 (2020): 554–61.

Fields, Howard L. "Setting the Stage for Pain: Allegorical Tales from Neuroscience." In *Pain and Its Transformations: The Interface of Biology and Culture*, edited by Sarah Coakley and Kay Kaufman Shelemay, 456p. Cambridge, MA: Harvard University Press, 2007.

François, B., E.M. Sternberg, and E. Fee. "The Lourdes Medical Cures Revisited." [In English]. *Journal of the History of Medicine and Allied Sciences* 69, no. 1 (2014): 135–62.

Gracely, R.H. "Clinician's Expectations Influence Placebo Analgesia." *Lancet* 1, no. 8419 (1985): 43.

Graham, Larry Kent. *Moral Injury: Restoring Wounded Souls*. Nashville: Abingdon Press, 2017.

---

[34]Ibid., 91.

Hauerwas, Stanley. "Suffering Presence: Twenty Five Years Later." In *Healing to All Their Flesh*, edited by Jeff Levin and Keith Meador, 242–58. Conshohocken, PA: Templeton Press, 2013.

Hróbjartsson, A., and P.C. Gøtzsche. "Is the Placebo Powerless?" *New England Journal of Medicine* 344, no. 21 (2001): 1594–602.

Hutchinson, Phil, and Daniel E. Moerman. "The Meaning Response, 'Placebo', and Methods." [In English]. *Perspectives in Biology and Medicine* 61, no. 3 (Summer 2018): 361–78.

Illueca, M., Y.S. Bradshaw, and D.B. Carr. "Spiritual Pain: A Symptom in Search of a Clinical Definition." *Journal of Religion and Health* 62, no. 3 (2023): 1920–32.

Illueca, M., and B.R. Doolittle. "The Use of Prayer in the Management of Pain: A Systematic Review." *Journal of Religion and Health* 59, no. 2 (2020): 681–99.

Kinghorn, Warren. "Combat Trauma and Moral Fragmentation: A Theological Account of Moral Injury." [In English]. *Journal of the Society of Christian Ethics* 32, no. 2 (2012): 57–74.

Luhrmann, T.M. *Of Two Minds: An Anthropologist Looks at American Psychiatry.* 1st Vintage Books ed. New York: Vintage Books, 2001.

Meints, S.M., M. Illueca, M.M. Miller, D. Osaji, and B. Doolittle. "The Pain and Prayer Scale (PPRAYERS): Development and Validation of a Scale to Measure Pain-Related Prayer." *Pain Medicine* 24, no. 7 (2023): 862–71.

Meints, S.M., C. Mosher, K.L. Rand, L. Ashburn-Nardo, and A.T. Hirsch. "An Experimental Investigation of the Relationships among Race, Prayer, and Pain." *Scandinavian Journal of Pain* 18, no. 3 (2018): 545–53.

Moerman, Daniel E. *Meaning, Medicine, and the "Placebo Effect".* Cambridge Studies in Medical Anthropology. Cambridge; New York: Cambridge University Press, 2002.

Nelson, Charles A., Nathan A. Fox, and Charles H. Zeanah. *Romania's Abandoned Children: Deprivation, Brain Development, and the Struggle for Recovery.* Cambridge, MA: Harvard University Press, 2014.

Pardo-Cabello, A.J., V. Manzano-Gamero, and E. Puche-Canas. "Placebo: A Brief Updated Review." *Naunyn Schmiedebergs Arch Pharmacol* 395, no. 11 (2022): 1343–56.

Raz, A., E. Raikhel, and R.D. Anbar. "Placebos in Medicine: Knowledge, Beliefs, and Patterns of Use." [In English]. *McGill Journal of Medicine* 11, no. 2 (2008): 206–11.

Van der Kolk, Bessel A. *The Body Keeps the Score: Brain, Mind, and Body in the Healing of Trauma.* New York: Viking, 2014.

Wolterstorff, Nicholas. *Lament for a Son.* Grand Rapids: Wm. B. Eerdmans Publishing, 1987.

5
Healing at the End

Chapter Outline	
Times to Die	90
Medicalized Death: A Failed Experiment	92
The Art of Dying	96
An Art of Dying	100
Working Together	102

Catherine wept in the church pew at the end of the service. We had just sung, "Nearer my God to Thee," an old gospel tune. The congregation had filed out to coffee hour. Alone she hunched in the same wooden pew where she had sat with Tony for decades. Tony had died three months before, after a protracted course of intestinal tumors. He had suffered. He was a church leader with a gregarious personality and strong opinions about everything. He wore loud red vests, sang hymns with gusto, and, for more than six decades, dearly, dearly loved his wife Catherine.

Before our eyes, he melted away, endured surgeries and chemo, and grew ever so weaker. The lively man grew quieter in church, shuffled home after worship exhausted. He would still smile, but with wistful, forlorn loss. He was dying. As a church, we visited him in the hospital, delivered meals to his home, prayed for him, and grieved alongside him. We loved him and Catherine as best we could, with the steady, awkward, sincere love that can only come from a close, small urban congregation. We had been down this path with others. We knew what to do.

Hope against hope, he perished on a sunny, wintry day, comfortable but numb with morphine. We were numb too. The funeral was a blur. In a new black dress, Catherine endured it all with sad smiles, polite niceties, and tears ever welling in her eyes. We laid him in the ground, ashes to ashes, dust to dust. Catherine taught us all about death: the persevering, steadfast love required to love someone from that first diagnosis, through the uncertainty and suffering of treatments, and to the final breath.

Three months later, as folks filed out of church, I asked Catherine, "Why are you crying?"

"That was Tony's favorite hymn. Whenever I hear it, I think of him. I realize now that he is dead. I guess I never realized it until now. He is really gone."

When does a person die? In Catherine's case, Tony's death occurred after he died. This often happens. The cycle of denial, anger, bargaining, grieving, and acceptance takes time and is not temporally related to the loved one's actual death. The process is often cyclical. "Nearer my God to Thee," triggered her realization of Tony's death.

There is the moment when the heart stops, when breath ceases, when the physician signs the death certificate. But death is more complicated than that. Death is a leave-taking. For some families, death occurs when their loved one suffers the irreversible stroke, when Alzheimer's leads to a nursing home, when the cancer ravages a body. The loved one's heart beats. The diaphragm contracts in breath. But, the loss has begun. Death can precede the moment the heart stops. It can even happen more than once.

Times to Die

When Lydia Dugdale was a young doctor, she met a man who died three times in the course of her hospital shift.[1] Mr. Turner was an elderly African American man with late stage cancer, in the midst of a renewed round of chemotherapy that Dugdale worried had already become more agony than treatment. When his heart stopped, she was part of the code team that revived him, cracking his frail ribs with CPR, putting him on a ventilator and moving him to intensive care. Within ninety minutes his heart stopped again. The revival process was repeated and again, somewhat to Dugdale's

---

[1] For what follows, see Chapter 1 "Death," in *The Lost Art of Dying: Reviving Forgotten Wisdom*, ed. Lydia S. Dugdale (New York: HarperOne, 2020).

chagrin, succeeded. Later still that same night, Mr. Turner died for the last time, despite a third round of medical efforts.

After Mr. Turner's first death, Dugdale had conferred with his daughters, gently asking if they would like to give instructions not to resuscitate their father if his heart stopped again. "No, Doctor," they responded. "We are Christians . . . We believe in miracles. You do whatever you can to keep him alive."[2] Medical care had proven it could literally raise the dead. But it had no hope of restoring Mr. Turner to the life his children sought.

Their response was not unusual. One study of spiritual support and medical care at the end of life found that patients with strong religious faith were on average *more* likely to opt for "heroic measures" and to maximize treatments with little likelihood of benefit.[3] Belief in miracles, the divine capacity to do the apparently impossible, is not here set in direct opposition to medical care, but instead encourages people to pursue its maximal, last ditch interventions. Medical marvels, like Dugdale's resuscitation efforts, are pursued not from any expectation they themselves can deliver the miraculous result but because they extend the time to hope for it.

This feature was noted to be particularly strong in minority populations that on average combine strong religious responses with the additional element of historical suspicions about fair treatment within medical institutions.[4] Resistance to allopathic medical treatment or prioritizing alternative forms of healing (from folk traditions or non-Western medical ones) can reflect both suspicion of the power imbalances in access to allopathic treatments and divergent understandings of health and healing.

The effectiveness of medical technology can turn death into an explicit decision point: when to take a patient off a ventilator, to remove external life support, or intravenous nutrition. Since few patients or families are well versed in the basis for a medical prognosis, there is always room for uncertainty about such decisions. In this way, the natural and inexorable event of death becomes something for which health professionals and loved ones must take responsibility, one more burden added to the final path.

---

[2]Ibid., 6.
[3]Andrea C. Phelps et al., "Religious Coping and Use of Intensive Life-Prolonging Care near Death in Patients with Advanced Cancer," *JAMA: The Journal of the American Medical Association* 301, no. 11 (2009): 1140–7.
[4]Tracy A. Balboni et al., "Provision of Spiritual Support to Patients with Advanced Cancer by Religious Communities and Associations with Medical Care at the End of Life," *JAMA Internal Medicine* 173, no. 12 (2013): 1109–17.

Catherine's story is about the full reality of death emerging long after the biological fact. Dr. Dugdale and Mr. Turner's story suggests that the biological fact may be delayed beyond the point when we could and should recognize its reality.

Medicalized Death: A Failed Experiment

Death is a boundary case in medicine. There is no treatment for it. There may be a blurred period, for a few moments following a cardiac arrest, for instance, where clinical death may possibly be reversed. But at the point at which such efforts cease, and a time of death is "called," the medical journey ends. For physicians whose practice is patient-facing, death is a constant companion.

It is both a sacred and a mundane moment. Some hospitals have adopted a practice for all in attendance at a death, particularly a "code death" marked by active measures, to pause together for a moment of silence.[5] This marks respect for the deceased person, and an important step in dealing with the trauma and distress of the medical staff. Nurses and doctors must maintain some emotional distance to do their work. But they also suffer the pain and loss before them. To simply tear off their gloves and walk on to the next thing may be inadequate to their own emotions, the pain of coming hard up against the wall beyond which they can do nothing.

At such a medically liturgical moment, it is as though a torch is passed. The body moves to another realm, one of "corpse care".[6] Even when a hospital bed is in great demand, some time is granted for the room of death to become a space for leave-taking, prayer or ritual, care for the body no longer aimed at reviving it but at restoring its natural aspect and dignity. From here on, it is religion and tradition that guide the treatment and preparation of the body, its washing and tending, its clothing, preparation, and final reception and disposition within communities of family, friendship and faith. The

---

[5] See "The Pause," https://thepause.me.
[6] Cody J. Sanders and Mikeal C. Parsons, *Corpse Care: Ethics for Tending the Dead* (Minneapolis, MN: Fortress Press, 2023).

healing tasks that remain are in support for the bereaved, in preserving memory, and in expressing hope for the future of the one who has died.

The mundane is never far from hand. In the emergency department, a doctor breaks the news of a loved one's death. Families ask if their loved one suffered, if more could have been done. There are tears, expressions of guilt, and then the awkward question, "What next?" The list is prosaic and long: calls to the funeral home and family members, an obituary to write, a funeral to plan. There are countless questions to answer. Open casket or closed? Cremation? Church or funeral home? Religious or secular service? Who will give the eulogy? Reception afterwards?

We have spoken so far, as our culture tends to, of death as an event and not of dying, a condition and a process. Historically, ministry and medicine were the two professions that involved intimate encounters with dying. It was a cardinal task for both ministers and physicians to prepare people for death and to accompany them through it. Both Christian spirituality and popular culture took the recollection of death as a necessary central theme. The meaningfulness of life's purposes and activities was measured from the perspective of its end. "*Momento mori*," a latin phrase meaning "remember that you must die," came to stand for a recurrent theme in literature, art, and religion from classical antiquity through early modern Christian culture. To contemplate one's death is to put things in their proper ultimate proportion.

Medicine lived most of its history frankly under the umbrella of mortality. Precisely because it could do little to prevent death, medicine gave its attention to tending the dying. The norm was "slow medicine," whose primary tools were prognosis and information about the course of the disease, stages on the way to death. These were tools that enabled the doctor to be a companion on the path and a guide for other companions. Knowledge about what is likely to happen (without great ability to change it) is a resource in making wise choices about the end of life, choices that are not only about pain and comfort, but about priorities and relationships.

In contexts drenched with expectation of death, people's outlooks were clearly different. "The necessity of nature's final victory was expected and accepted in generations before our own. Doctors were far more willing to recognize the signs of defeat and far less arrogant about denying them."[7] We are not talking about ancient history. Lewis Thomas, who did his internship

---

[7] Sherwin B. Nuland, *How We Die: Reflections on Life's Final Chapter*, 1st ed. (New York: A.A. Knopf: Distributed by Random House, Inc., 1994), 259.

in 1937, reports that even at that time "If being in a hospital bed made a difference, it was mostly the difference produced by warmth, shelter, and food and attentive, friendly care . . . Whether you survived or not depended on the natural history of the disease itself. Medicine made little or no difference."[8] One of the things this meant is that people gave more thought to a "good death." In our setting the term has a kind of oxymoronic character. Where such a concern exists, it is more likely to stem from patients than from doctors, though doctors are more likely to have concrete knowledge of the relevant data.

In only a few generations, antibiotics, surgical expertise, and pharmaceutical discoveries have reversed Thomas' perspective. Mortality increasingly became a guilty shadow within the realm of healing. Rather than a normal staple of any medical practice, death has acquired a certain taint of failure, an embarrassment to the default expectation for cure and recovery. Indeed, new branches of medicine now treat mortality itself as a disease, and seek to extend longevity in perpetuity.

In many ways a blessing, this state of affairs has made the process of dying a medical orphan. Medicine came increasingly to view the dying person as a patient and, as such always a candidate for additional treatment. The proliferation of silos in medicine exacerbates this problem, as specialists emphasize the benefits of their own strategies, and no one claims the task of counsel regarding overall cost/benefit. Studies show that oncologists, for instance, often do not initiate "end of life conversations" with patients until literally the final days. In medical school, there are workshops to teach future physicians how to break bad news with sensitivity. There are lectures that teach how to fill out the death certificate, and when to call the state coroner. Without a picture of a good death as a positive, healing outcome, it is no surprise that doctors have been given fewer resources to achieve it.

In this sense, health care workers now bear a spiritual burden their ancestors did not. It is their job to come up with every possible strategy to overcome death. They must be the "devil's advocate" who seeks out every avenue of healing, no matter how painful, for they have the specialized knowledge and means to do so. The surgeon Sherwin Nuland says, "Of all the professions, medicine is the one most likely to attract people with high

---

[8]Lewis Thomas, *The Youngest Science: Notes of a Medicine-Watcher* (Oxford; New York: Oxford University Press, 1985), 40.

personal anxieties about dying."[9] If this true, then we are the beneficiaries of their burden. We want them to be advocates of medical hope, to leave no stone unturned in offering options, to be obsessive for life. But that role sits uneasily with the task of assessing the downside of treatments, of judging not the marginal effect of a drug regimen on some biological marker, but the wisest course for a dying patient's well-being. It is difficult to disentangle treatment from care, to turn from the technological and to turn toward human presence to the patient.

We are well acquainted with the statistics that indicate the large proportion of a lifetime's medical expenditures that occur within months of death. Atul Gawande notes, as a surgeon, that the most common week in which surgery occurs in a person's life is the last week. The most common day is their final day.[10] This suggests not only the limited utility of surgery in those particular cases, but the high treatment context of such deaths.

In the United States, death is highly medicalized. Only 31 percent of deaths occur at home (though this number has been slowly rising), with the rest in hospitals (35 percent), nursing homes (27 percent), or elsewhere (7 percent) [11] Many obituaries hopefully report that the deceased "died quietly at home, surrounded by family and friends." Is this the right model? Increasingly, families realize that caring for a dying family member is difficult. Often, family members are put in the difficult position of addressing pain, bodily functions, cleaning, and feeding, as well as managing forms of medical care that are recent developments. Dying is hard work—emotionally and physically demanding—for the one dying and for their care givers. While we may aspire to the peaceful death at home, we (both as patients and as medical workers) are ambivalent about the path that leads there. We often have the means and the will to treat the finality of our condition as one more medical crisis to be overcome, at least temporarily. In such a crisis, medical interventions may be at their most intensive and extreme.

As Gawande wrote in his book *Being Mortal,* "This experiment of making mortality a medical experience is just decades old. It is young. And the

---

[9] Nuland, *How We Die: Reflections on Life's Final Chapter,* 258.
[10] See Finlay Young, "Atul Gawande: The Smiling Angel of a Happy Death," *Newsweek,* 2014.
[11] Sarah H. Cross and Haider J. Warraich, "Changes in the Place of Death in the United States," *New England Journal of Medicine* 381, no. 24 (2019): 2369–70.

evidence is that it is failing."[12] It fails patients: the elderly and terminally ill endure debilitating treatments and institutions of care that combine to cut them off prematurely from the things that truly matter to them. It fails doctors as well. Gawande confesses that he wrote his book because his dead and dying patients haunted his dreams. Although his entire career was animated by satisfaction at solving difficult problems, he realized he lacked any coherent vision of "how people might live successfully all the way to their very end."[13]

He rediscovered, like a kind of conversion, what his ancestors in the medical field had known of necessity: "some of the most gratifying moments in my practice now come from feeling more confident with people who have unfixable problems, and trying to understand how to help them navigate through," to decide what priorities we are actually chasing.[14]

The Art of Dying

Religious faith and communities would appear obvious reference points for a vision of death that could correct and enrich a purely medical perspective. Such faith typically addresses death directly with convictions about meaning and purpose that transcend mortal life and articulate values that can relativize medical "success." Ideally, one can imagine a seamless transition from a medical orientation prioritizing cure toward an existential orientation prioritizing a meaningful end of life. Obstacles to such a transition are not found only in the tension between the medical and the religious approaches, but within religion itself.

Today, extensive consideration of death is likely to appear morbid, and to the extent that people give consideration to a good death, it is likely to be defined primarily in technocratic terms, by absence of pain (and the active use of medications to avoid both physical and emotional distress) and by prior logistical planning (having put one's affairs in order in such a way as to clarify things for caregivers and to avoid any burden on survivors). So the "art of dying" actively recognized in medical circles has come to be identified

---

[12]Atul Gawande, *Being Mortal: Medicine and What Matters in the End*, 1st Picador ed. (India: Penguin Books, 2014), 9.
[13]Ibid.
[14]Quoted in Young, "Atul Gawande: The Smiling Angel of a Happy Death."

with advance directives and health care proxy arrangements. These are valuable tools, and they do address situations where doctors feel legally compelled to persist in treatments that they believe are useless or intensify and prolong suffering. But such preparations often prove fruitless because of miscommunication in medical settings.

Religious communities have often responded to this widening gap in the medical world's approach to dying, not with a compensatory emphasis and attention on it, but with a parallel deemphasis. The prevalence of "memento mori" in spiritual reflection and ecclesial life in the past had a large empirical component. It was recognition, not imposition, of a consideration that could never be far from anyone's daily experience. In the new medical world, the theme of death could appear morbid or even a kind of special pleading, wielding the possible imminence of death as a threat to compel people to get right with God. Many clergy, rightly, seek to underline the significance of religious conviction for faithful living and social transformation here and now, and not merely as an "insurance policy" for life after death. But it is unfortunate if this leads the church to back away from offering the very insight and preparation that are more essential than ever to leaven the medicalization of mortality.

During the Covid-19 pandemic, our culture was forced into collective contemplation of our mortality. In our societies, death has been for some time an individual event. The absence of fear of mass death means the absence of common reflection on it. Ash Wednesday, with its ritual recall that "from ashes you came and to ashes you will return," once concretized a thought that could rarely have been far from the mind of those surrounded with death on every side. Today, it is an odd outlier. The extraordinary outpouring of public emotion around some celebrity deaths (Princess Diana, for instance) reflects in part a response to the rare opportunity for collective attention to mortality.

Christian faith had since its beginnings included pastoral preparation for death and care for the dying. Its spread was bound up with the message of the resurrection of Christ and the coordinate hope for followers to participate in that resurrection. For believers, as for Christ, death was the necessary gateway to that hope. Though early Christian writers celebrated liberation from the fear of death, they neither cultivated a philosophical indifference to it nor did they downplay its gravity. Some versions of early Christianity understood Jesus to have been translated directly to heaven without suffering death at all and saw the soul as a deathless spirit untouched by the fate of the body.¹⁵ But these were not the views that prevailed. Jesus truly died a brutal death, as biologically definitive as that of all of his followers. The path of faith lay through this fact and not around it.

One effect of the devastating waves of plague in medieval Europe was the rise of a new "do-it-yourself" literature for preparation for death. People had seen that one could not always expect religious leaders or physicians to be on hand in such extreme conditions. The model for many of these manuals on the "art of dying" came from a work by Jean Gerson, a famous French theologian.¹⁶ Later handbooks, eventually produced by Catholics, Lutherans, Calvinists, and Anglicans alike, shared the same basic elements. These included a "commendation" of death (in the sense of indicating the salutary benefits that can come from facing up to death's unavoidable challenge), a warning about the temptations for the dying and how to resist these, a short rehearsal of Christian beliefs for spiritual reassurance, and instructions on the imitation of Christ and on specific prayers to be said by the dying person and by those who cared for them.

This set a pattern that, in a simplified and generically Protestant form, became a widespread cultural theme in the United States.¹⁷ Recognizing the imminence of death, a person accepted this reality with regret but resignation. They came to terms with family and friends, offering and receiving forgiveness. They would confess their sins and commend their souls to God. A "good death" was one which gave opportunity for all of these elements to be played out. It was one which did not take a person totally unaware, one to which the dying person came having made peace with their neighbors and with God. Such a view of death frankly acknowledged the unavoidable elements of suffering: the intrinsic anguish of separation and grief, the pain of bodily decay and dysfunction, the loss of skills and capacities, and the extreme dependence on the care of others. But it focused on what remained possible in the final days and hours.

The good death became the standard against which other forms of death were judged. There are tragic and unjust deaths, those that come to the very

---

¹⁵Such was the view of some later designated as Gnostic Christians. See Bentley Layton and David Brakke, *The Gnostic Scriptures*, 2nd ed., The Anchor Yale Bible Reference Library (New Haven, CT: Yale University Press, 2021).

¹⁶For what follows in this paragraph, see Allen Verhey, *The Christian Art of Dying: Learning from Jesus* (Grand Rapids, MI: William B. Eerdmans Pub., 2011). 85–7.

¹⁷See the summary in ibid., 11. See also Drew Gilpin Faust, *This Republic of Suffering: Death and the American Civil War*, 1st ed. (New York: Alfred A. Knopf, 2008).

young or ones that are preventable or accidental (including for instance those that are the result of medical mistakes), or that were maliciously abetted or inflicted. In such cases, there is moral pain or insult added to the unavoidable fact. And there are qualities that unequivocally characterize a "bad death:" extreme physical pain, intense emotional distress, isolation or estrangement from community support, loss of hope.

So familiar was this pattern for a good death that it became a kind of cliché: pious deathbed scenes and last minute conversions became standard sentimental conventions in literature and religion. The good death became a stereotype, too good to be true. Charles Dickens did not mean his account of the edifying death of his virtuous child heroine, little Nell, in *The Old Curiosity Shop* as satire. But many readers of a later time would have agreed with the statement attributed to Oscar Wilde: "One must have a heart of stone to read the death of little Nell without laughing." This indicated that the expectation of a good death could become an oppressive script more than a spiritual support.

Many of those who suffer through a slow decline through disease are heard to say that dying is harder than death. Adjunct to our medicalization of death is a desire to limit the suffering attached to it. The last thing we want to add to the pain of illness and the prospect of death is to burden the dying person with tasks or expectations we prescribe for their own supposed good, or only in order to satisfy the needs of others around them. But not all such concerns are imposed from the outside. There are internal "tasks" defined by a person's own hopes and commitments, and we cannot die in isolation from our relationships any more than we can live so.

Contemporary people may be scandalized at the prospect of Christian encouragement of self-examination and spiritual preparation for an eschatological judgment or with Buddhist prescriptions for elaborate programs of meditation and imagery to be carried out by the dying person to assure a better rebirth. These look like a burden of gratuitous performance anxiety layered onto someone's final days. And so they may be, where there is no organic connection for the dying person. But for most of human history, it was hardly so. In the Christian tradition, the art of dying was not seen as an "over and above" obligation laid upon people at the end of life, but a consoling wisdom to guide someone through unavoidable parts of the experience of dying: fear, despair, anger, pain.

It was a prescription, of sorts, to treat the "co-morbidities" of death. These include regret and guilt about our past, the suffering of lost hopes and aspirations, burning desires for forgiveness, reconciliation, or for achievements still possible in this life, fears for those we leave behind and perhaps for our own future state, hope for peace in letting go. It is a terrible message to convey to the dying that they can "do it wrong," and so increase other people's pain, or lose religious rewards. But a good death means that there are things that can go right, even in the midst of pain and loss, and that the dignity of the dying requires us to think about those things.

A good death in those terms presupposed time and opportunity for these things, a space of time that was clearly recognized as "dying." This is something in shorter supply in our world, both because much that led to lingering death in the past can now be treated and because we tend not to place someone in the category of "dying" rather than "under treatment" until the last possible moment. This means that if the art of dying is to be relevant today, some of its features probably have to be included in our normal lives as preparatory.

An Art of Dying

What would this look like? Lydia Dugdale offers some precious glimpses in her book *The Lost Art of Dying*.[18] As a doctor, she says it is important to ask doctors questions that address what is truly important for the dying. Not "What is the success rate with this operation?" but "What are the most likely downsides that go with the operation and what is the recovery likely to be like?" Not "Might this medicine help?" but "Have you ever seen this drug help someone with my form of cancer?" or even better "How likely is it that this treatment to leave me unable to enjoy (and here the question must be very individual) food, or knitting, or online conversation with family, as I am still currently able to do?"

From the medical side, many practitioners are beginning to emphasize patient assessments that look beyond narrow statistical measures for the outcome of specific procedures toward more realistic perspectives on the likely life course results. A "successful" surgery or chemotherapy regimen may produce the advertised reduction in tumor size or even in extended survival, while it may also reliably be associated with precipitous declines in other aspects of health that mean more to the patient. Assessing patients for

---

[18]For the following paragraph, see Dugdale, *The Lost Art of Dying: Reviving Forgotten Wisdom*, 190.

"frailty" would be an example.[19] Such evaluation takes into account many factors to determine not just whether, say, an elderly person is likely to survive their time in the operating room for a particular procedure (the probability may be very high), but whether their recovery trajectory will restore them, even briefly, to the quality of life they enjoyed at the time of the procedure (the probability may be very low).

To be able to ask questions with such specificity requires not only an appreciation for medical complexity but self-knowledge, recognition of the things we truly value about our own lives. The medieval manuals focused on the temptations of dying—temptations like impatience, pride, greed—and the virtues that countered them. These seem to us perhaps like extrinsic concerns, an injunction to be moral while dying. But Dugdale's discussion makes clear that the virtues in question: patience, humility, faith, "letting go," are in fact deeply germane for dying well.

The impatience for medicine to provide a cure, the greed to have everything (every capacity, every security, every opportunity) as long as possible—these things can rapidly become counter-productive. Specifically, they can actually rob us of the greatest quality of life in our dying. It is the lack of such virtues that incline us to run headlong toward every medical option possible. The self-examination the art of dying commends aims not at self-mortification or fulfilment of some wooden ideal, but at clarity about what matters to us. Such clarity is the only basis for negotiating the medical thicket that may attend our dying. It equips us (and those around us) to say "no" to some things in the service of priorities we have identified and learned to practice . . . and also "yes" to some of the wonderful palliative and supportive resources of medicine when oriented in this way.

These virtues are broader than specific religious traditions, but they are concretely formulated and supported within religious communities, where they are integral to a wider set of values and aims. They are also not limited to an intellectual level, as in beliefs about what matters to us. They exist in embodied forms, such as in corporate singing. There are benefits to corporate singing that may be further enhanced when it embodies specific religious content. Dugdale recounts the story of a woman with advanced dementia who had long been incommunicative. When a visitor began to play "Amazing

---

[19] See for instance Dae Hyun Kim and Kenneth Rockwood, "Frailty in Older Adults," *New England Journal of Medicine* 391, no. 6 (2024): 538–48.

Grace" on the violin, the woman sang along.[20] We have a former student, a choir director, who has studied the health benefits of singing together, and another who now focuses specifically on the role of music in support for dying people.

Virtues for dying are best cultivated far ahead of time. Indeed, they serve human flourishing in life as much as at the end of it. This is why Gawande's study of the medical treatment of death branched out to spend as much time exploring the living conditions of healthy elderly people as exploring end-of-life decision making.[21] He contrasts the elderly resident on the slopes of Mt. St. Helen who refused to be moved from his home and perished in the volcano's explosion with a resident he met in a retirement home who felt entombed in an alien and sterile environment. Gawande lamented a world where the choices seemed to be "going down with the volcano or yielding all control over our lives."[22]

Retirement communities or care homes seek to balance the safety of their residents with their freedom and life goals. The orphanage infants at the dawn of life we discussed earlier, who had all of life's basic needs but failed to flourish without love, are a kind of mirror image of elderly or health-restricted residents in care facilities engineered for safety (and provider convenience) who wither and fail from the inability to maintain activities that keep life meaningful. Those activities can range from the capacity to keep a pet to the right to lock one's door. What makes life worth living, in terms of concrete daily activities, is a prescription that needs to be written by the patient, and then coordinated with the medical plan. This is a crucial lesson for the dying and their loved ones, but it applies much more widely.

Working Together

The end of life arena is one where the mutuality in the relation of faith and medicine seems most evident to people in both religious and medical communities. The synergy is one of careful consideration about what medical resources can most effectively be used to serve supportive and not curative

---

[20]Dugdale, *The Lost Art of Dying: Reviving Forgotten Wisdom*, 212.
[21]See for instance Chapter Four "Assistance," in Gawande, *Being Mortal: Medicine and What Matters in the End*.
[22]Ibid., 68.

ends, active affirmation of the spiritual meaning the dying person wishes to bring to their experience, and cultivation of the community connections that can undergird that path. Medical schools routinely recognize spirituality as a significant feature in end of life care, even if the clinical implementation of that recognition is often wanting. Palliative care increasingly is part of standard medical education. At Yale, a required module on palliative care brings together medical and nursing students with students from the divinity school and the school of social work to reflect together on a case study in end of life care. In the divinity school, a significant number of clergy prepare to make hospice chaplaincy one of their specialties, and prospective parish clergy train in many of the same skills.

There has in fact been a revival of concern for a "good death," signified most notably by the modern hospice movement founded by Cicely Saunders. A conscious attempt to recover both the Christian ideal of the art of dying and the institutional form of the monastic hospice for the sick, this movement sought to differentiate supportive care from purely medical care. It prioritized quality of life, community support, and conscious acceptance of a "time to die." Saunders' hospice in London had two explicit dimensions. The first was specifically medical. It was the development and application of medical resources for "palliation," not to cure the disease but to alleviate all the physical symptoms of dying. The second was specifically Christian. It was to reclaim human hospitality and spiritual support as the context for the end of life.

The hospice movement has grown to serve a pluralistic population, and on the whole, it has maintained a sensitivity to the spiritual dimension of its task in continuity with Saunders' vision. This marks it out as a bright spot in the integration of the medical and the religious. There is certainly room for religious groups to continue to innovate in their own ways in this space. One student in our class belonged to a circle of friends who had long dreamed of forming an intentional community whose centerpiece would be providing health care in a holistic and spiritually grounded setting. After graduation, she became chaplain at a large, church-related retirement community, and started a small religious community whose special vocation included the development of hospice care for those within the retirement community. The hope was that by building relationships with residents over years, the community would help prepare them for the end of life, and would be able to support and accompany them through their seasons of death. When such retirement facilities advertise to prospective residents, they regularly emphasize their recreational and community resources, their food services, the availability of increasing levels of medical care. It is rare, even in church related facilities, to see one that advertises its hospice services, its vision for a good death. But from both medical and spiritual perspectives, this makes extremely good sense, a frank encouragement for the "art of dying."

In intensive attempts at cure—challenging chemotherapy regimes, transplants and surgeries with long recovery arcs—patients and their families often enter a kind of ascetic struggle, a "dark night" marked by pain, emotional devastation, relational stress. This investment is made in hopes of renewed life and recovery. Hospice care and the palliative medicine it practices reverse the polarities. Everything is done in the interests of spiritual well-being, preservation of normal pleasures of food or sensation or conversation, and freedom from pain, even at the cost of duration of life. This transition—from a thoroughly medical outlook to one in which the resources of medicine are used for an end whose nature is not primarily medical—is not an easy one to negotiate. This is represented by the fact that a patient's entry into hospice care often requires paperwork recognizing a departure from medicine as usual.

This is ironic because the boundaries in experience are not so clear cut. A study randomly assigned patients with advanced forms of lung cancer (and so poor prognoses for survival) into two groups.[23] One group, from the very time of first diagnosis, received a full range of palliative care resources, including access to chaplains and social workers and hospice-type preparations. The other group was addressed with standard medical options, until such time as those patients might request consideration of palliative care. Those in the first group showed less depression, opted less often for chemotherapy treatments, and opted less often for aggressive end of life measures. In addition to better reported quality of life, those in the first group on average actually lived two and a half months longer than those under purely medical treatment (and this when the life expectancy at diagnosis was itself measured in months).

Another study found that two-thirds of cancer patients with a terminal diagnosis had no conversations with their doctors about their aims in end of life care.[24] Those who did have such conversations opted for less aggressive

---

[23] Jennifer S.M.D. Temel et al., "Early Palliative Care for Patients with Metastatic Non-Small-Cell Lung Cancer," *The New England Journal of Medicine* 363, no. 8 (2010): 733–42.
[24] Alexi A. Wright et al., "Associations between End-of-Life Discussions, Patient Mental Health, Medical Care near Death, and Caregiver Bereavement Adjustment," *JAMA* 300, no. 14 (2008): 1665–73.

measures and reported better quality of life. In follow up with family and loved ones after the patient's death, those associated with the conversation patients showed less traumatic bereavement. One way to look at this data is to note that those who were, from the beginning of their life-threatening diagnosis, encouraged to reflect directly on their mortality, died, and lived, more successfully than those that focused only on combating that mortality. The creation of palliative care as its own specialty has been a major step forward, but its virtues should not be isolated from the rest of medicine.

References

Balboni, Tracy A., Michael Balboni, Andrea C. Enzinger, Kathleen Gallivan, M. Elizabeth Paulk, Alexi Wright, Karen Steinhauser, Tyler J. VanderWeele, and Holly G. Prigerson. "Provision of Spiritual Support to Patients with Advanced Cancer by Religious Communities and Associations with Medical Care at the End of Life." *JAMA Internal Medicine* 173, no. 12 (2013): 1109–17.

Cross, Sarah H., and Haider J. Warraich. "Changes in the Place of Death in the United States." *New England Journal of Medicine* 381, no. 24 (2019): 2369–70.

Dugdale, Lydia S. *The Lost Art of Dying: Reviving Forgotten Wisdom*. New York: HarperOne, 2020.

Faust, Drew Gilpin. *This Republic of Suffering: Death and the American Civil War*. 1st ed. New York: Alfred A. Knopf, 2008.

Gawande, Atul. *Being Mortal: Medicine and What Matters in the End*. First Picador ed. India: Penguin Books, 2014.

Kim, Dae Hyun, and Kenneth Rockwood. "Frailty in Older Adults." *New England Journal of Medicine* 391, no. 6 (2024): 538–48.

Layton, Bentley, and David Brakke. *The Gnostic Scriptures*. The Anchor Yale Bible Reference Library. 2nd ed. ed. New Haven, CT: Yale University Press, 2021.

Nuland, Sherwin B. *How We Die: Reflections on Life's Final Chapter*. 1st ed. New York: A.A. Knopf : Distributed by Random House, Inc., 1994.

Phelps, Andrea C., Paul K. Maciejewski, Matthew Nilsson, Tracy A. Balboni, Alexi A. Wright, M. Elizabeth Paulk, Elizabeth Trice, et al. "Religious Coping and Use of Intensive Life-Prolonging Care near Death in Patients with Advanced Cancer." [In English]. *JAMA: The journal of the American Medical Association* 301, no. 11 (2009): 1140–7.

Sanders, Cody J., and Mikeal C. Parsons. *Corpse Care: Ethics for Tending the Dead*. Minneapolis, MN: Fortress Press, 2023.

Temel, Jennifer S.M.D., Joseph A. PhD Greer, Alona M.A. Muzikansky, Emily R.R.N. Gallagher, Sonal M.B.B.S.M.P.H. Admane, Vicki A.M.D.M.P.H. Jackson, Constance M.A.P.N. Dahlin, et al. "Early Palliative Care for Patients with Metastatic Non-Small-Cell Lung Cancer." [In English]. *The New England Journal of Medicine* 363, no. 8 (2010): 733–42.

Thomas, Lewis. *The Youngest Science: Notes of a Medicine-Watcher*. Oxford; New York: Oxford University Press, 1985.

Verhey, Allen. *The Christian Art of Dying : Learning from Jesus*. Grand Rapids, MI: William B. Eerdmans Pub., 2011.

Wright, Alexi A., Baohui Zhang, Alaka Ray, Jennifer W. Mack, Elizabeth Trice, Tracy Balboni, Susan L. Mitchell, et al. "Associations between End-of-Life Discussions, Patient Mental Health, Medical Care near Death, and Caregiver Bereavement Adjustment." *JAMA* 300, no. 14 (2008): 1665–73.

Young, Finlay. "Atul Gawande: The Smiling Angel of a Happy Death." *Newsweek*, 2014, online article.

6

Is Religion Good For You?

Chapter Outline	
The Revolution in Research on Religion and Health	109
Webs of Truth, Webs of Meaning	113
Next Steps in Research	117
Confounders	119
Integration	124

What is more effective than cholesterol-lowering medications to prolong your life? The answer: religious participation.[1] If religious participation could be packaged as a drug, judged by the same criteria that the Federal Drug Administration uses, it would dwarf the impact of Lipitor or Prozac. This is not only news to most people. It is likely to strike them as a strange conjunction of categories. Indeed, both religious and non-religious people may wonder how faith could function as a medication. Health effects constitute only a part of religion as a whole, but they are a key meeting point in the conversation between theology and medicine.

That dialogue involves a plunge into statistics and epidemiology. This is the language evidence-based medicine uses to explore whether religion is good for your health (and if so, perhaps even to explore what *kinds* of religion are most often so). At Yale Medical School, quantitative data drives the conversation. This is a good thing, for randomized controlled trials, prospective cohort studies, and big data crunches save lives. Empirical

---

[1] Daniel E. Hall, "Religious Attendance: More Cost-Effective Than Lipitor?" *Journal of the American Board of Family Medicine* 19, no. 2 (2006): 103–9.

research brought us insulin and antibiotics, chemotherapy, and vaccines. We practice sterile technique in delivering newborns so mothers and infants do not die from sepsis. We no longer bleed people to re-adjust their humors. The scientific method has rescued us from superstition and harmful practices.

Up the street at Yale Divinity School, ethics, theology, and history drive the conversation. Truth is discerned in the flow of thinkers, traditions, and religious experience over time. Regression analysis and big data do not figure as heavily as qualitative and analytical discussion. Art, literature, and music are part of the conversation. This too is a good thing. Philosophical and moral reflection have improved our lives. Religious and humanistic perspectives remind us that data do not speak for themselves. We now reject the assumptions of standard medical practice that diagnosed runaway slaves with a mental disease ("Drapetomania") or allowed the Tuskegee syphilis scandals, or scientifically justified the application of eugenics in public health, or prescribed the warehousing of the developmentally and mentally disabled.[2] These changes were not driven by randomized control trials and peer reviewed research, but by reinterpretations of our normative beliefs and social movements. Religious and moral insight has sometimes rescued us from medical arrogance and medical abuses.

Just as religious people do not typically speak the language of statistical tests, so scientists do not typically speak the language of reconciliation, justice, or forgiveness. This is, on the whole a healthy division of labor. But the data perspective can stimulate theology to be more rigorous and grounded. Theological perspectives can stimulate medical science to ask a wider range of questions and to reflect critically on the assumptions it brings to producing and interpreting its data.

During the Covid-19 pandemic, we lived through a very public immersion in this discourse of randomized control trials and epidemiological evidence. Controversy over what it meant to "follow the science" turned upon debate over what constituted valid evidence, which in turn depended upon which recent studies about the virus, vaccines, and public health best met the methodological standards for such research. Professionals and lay people alike were trying to trace the line from research to practice in real time. In all

---

[2] On Drapetomania, see Loren Schweninger, "Counting the Costs: Southern Planters and the Problem of Runaway Slaves, 1790–1860," *Business and Economic History* 28, no. 2 (1999): 267–75.

of the specific topics treated in this book, that methodological concern is part of the backdrop.

Many religious people resist addressing religion in a statistical or quantitative way, convinced that such an approach misses what is most important: the lived, immediate, and personal quality of faith and its practices. They may also fear that religious practices will be judged and found wanting. For if one turns to such study for validation of religion's role in health, one must be willing to accept also evidence for negative effects. Many doctors and medical researchers ignore religion as a variable in their research or practice on the assumption that it cannot contribute anything substantive by way of causal effects or health outcomes. Bridging this gap requires people who are fluent in, and appreciative of, both languages.

The Revolution in Research on Religion and Health

Research bearing on spiritual effects on health has a longer history and a greater depth of peer-reviewed publication than is generally recognized in the medical arena. Figures otherwise legendary in the history of medicine often showed an interest in this topic that is tacitly excised from their legacies. For instance, a pioneer of modern scientific medicine, William Osler, published a famous article, "The Faith that Heals," in the British Medical Journal in 1910.[3] As medicine became a laboratory-based scientific discipline, the cultural conflict between science and religion became more marked. Though many medical institutions existed in religious settings, and despite the historically close associations of ministry and healing, religion became a somewhat taboo topic in medical research. By the middle of the twentieth century, the subject was in eclipse. The research that did exist had become largely invisible.

David Larson was one of those who changed this trajectory. During Larson's training as a psychiatrist in the 1970s, he reported that religion was mentioned only as a pathology.[4] Religion was a "borderline psychosis . . . a

---

[3] William Osler, "The Faith That Heals," *BMJ (Online)* 1, no. 2581 (1910): 1470–2.
[4] Interview with David Larson, https://www.faithandhealthconnection.org/wp-content/uploads/2007/11/insight-on-the-news-david-larson-interview.pdf.

regression, an escape, a projection on the world of a primitive infantile state," reported the Group for the Advancement of Psychiatry.[5] When he founded the National Institute for Healthcare Research in 1991 to serve as a clearing house for study of spirituality and health, he estimated only three medical schools then offered any course on the topic.[6]

Establishment of a field of academic research on religious factors in health and medical care is the accomplishment of a generation of pioneering figures such as Larson, Jeff Levin, and Harold Koenig.[7] Larson's contribution was cut short by his untimely death in 2002, but his story is representative. In the face of indifference or even hostility from his scholarly and medical peers, Larson insisted on treating religious practice as a serious variable in medical research.[8] To this end, he led the development of a now-standard research methodology, the systematic review. Larson undertook a painstaking investigation of all the good quality studies in the existing psychiatric research literature that contained information on religion as a variable.

In a public talk, he remembered that he set out with the hypothesis that religious people would prove to be "no crazier than anyone else."[9] That is, he expected the data to have a bell curve distribution, with equally small "tails" at either end of the distribution, representing studies suggesting either negative or positive relations, while the bulk of the studies would be in the middle, showing no significant effect either way. In fact, he found that some 80 percent of the data indicated a beneficial link between religion and health[10]. This result was all the more impressive, as the primary data had been assembled "blind," since the authors gathering it had no intention to test this hypothesis. The fruit of the work of Larson and many others is a rich and growing base of research, epitomized in the massive *Handbook of*

---

[5] Arthur J. Deikman, "Review of Mysticism: Spiritual Quest or Psychic Disorder?" *Journal of Nervous and Mental Disease* 165 (1977): 214.
[6] By 1999, half of medical schools did. Today it is the absence of such courses that is rare.
[7] See the bibliography for works by Koenig and Levin. Both have conducted research in their own rights. Koenig heads up the premier research program in this field at Duke University. Levin is the author of a major historical review of religion and medicine.
[8] David B. Larson and Susan S. Larson, *The Forgotten Factor in Physical and Mental Health: What Does the Research Show?: An Independent Study Seminar* (Rockville, MD: National Institute for Healthcare, 1994).
[9] Heim's recollection from attendance at Larson's talk. See also Susan S. Larson, "David: My Daring, Dauntless, Devoted White Knight," in *Faith, Medicine, and Science: A Festschrift in Honor of Dr. David B. Larson*, ed. David B. Larson, Jeffrey S. Levin, and Harold G. Koenig (Binghamton, NY: Haworth Pastoral Press, 2005), 230.
[10] Larson, Levin, and Koenig, *Faith, Medicine, and Science: A Festschrift in Honor of Dr. David B. Larson*, 230–1.

Religion and Health, now edited by Harold Koenig, which catalogs research relevant to religion in virtually every dimension of health.[11]

The situation today is quite the reverse of that which Larson originally encountered. The number of studies in the area continues to multiply. And scholarly literature today generally presumes an empirically established positive correlation between religious participation and physical well-being.[12] That correlation holds across an impressive range of medical indicators, as varied as viral load in HIV, pulmonary function in cystic fibrosis, completed suicide, biological risk factors for coronary artery disease, likelihood to smoke cigarettes, lifetime incidence of depression.[13]

We can illustrate with one impressive recent project, which recruited 120 different teams to run studies in different parts of the world on the relation between religious outlook and reported well-being, using a variety of analytical methods.[14] The design of the project was intended to avoid the effect of bias in any individual researcher or any individual technique. All but three teams reported a statistically significant positive result. Prior to the study, and then subsequent to reviewing its results, the individual researchers involved were asked about their assessments of this proposition: "How likely do you think it is that religiosity is related to higher self-reported well-being?" A strong majority began with a positive view of this relation (based on their reading of prior research). After reviewing the data, that majority grew (85 percent had a positive assessment and only 3 percent thought the relation unlikely) and a large majority also moved further toward the "very likely" end of a seven point spectrum, where "very unlikely" was at the other extreme.[15]

There are, of course, also negative findings, which indicate correlations where religious affiliation or practice has no effect on health or where some types of religious orientation are associated with worse outcomes. One

---

[11]See Harold G. Koenig, Dana E. King, and Verna Benner Carson, *Handbook of Religion and Health*, 2nd ed. (Oxford; New York: Oxford University Press, 2012); David H. Rosmarin and Harold G. Koenig, *Handbook of Spirituality, Religion, and Mental Health*, 2nd ed. (London; San Diego, CA: Academic Press, an imprint of Elsevier, 2020); Koenig, King, and Carson, *Handbook of Religion and Health*.
[12]For two representative surveys see Suzanne Hoogeveen et al., "A Many-Analysts Approach to the Relation between Religiosity and Well-Being," *Religion, Brain & Behavior* 13, no. 3 (2023): 237–83; Harold G.M.D. Koenig, "Religion, Spirituality, and Health: A Review and Update," *Advances in Mind-Body Medicine* 29, no. 3 (2015): 19–26.
[13]For this list, see "Religion, Spirituality, and Health: A Review and Update."
[14]Hoogeveen et al., "A Many-Analysts Approach to the Relation between Religiosity and Well-Being."
[15]Ibid., 249–50. 11 percent were neutral.

researcher who explored this question is Gail Ironson, who explored perceptions of God and health benefits. Those who believe in a benevolent God, a Creator who extends love and forgiveness, tend to be happier and have improved health outcomes. Those who believe in a malevolent, punishing God tend to do worse.[16]

Even a practice as apparently benign as mindfulness meditation proves, upon examination, to have downsides as well as benefits. Mindfulness is a powerful technique with a rich religious tradition, particularly in Buddhism and Hinduism, as well as Western monasticism. It may be the outstanding contemporary example of a synergistic blending of the medical and the spiritual. It has proven helpful to many, associated with relaxation, improved stress hormone levels, and concentration.[17]

A Brown psychologist, Willoughby Britton, was led by some individual anecdotes to investigate possible negative effects of meditation. She discovered that the numerous studies of the benefits of meditation had virtually never offered their participants an opportunity to register any negative experiences. When she simply included questions on this topic, she was surprised to see that many reported distressing outcomes, at the extreme including hospitalization and incapacitation.[18]

She subsequently formed a "Dark Night" project to study the negative results of meditation practice and a "Do No Harm" educational program to inform meditation teachers.[19] Britton pointed out that such destructive possibilities were well recognized in the Buddhist texts that were often the inspiration for these practices. That wisdom had been strained out of awareness as meditation instruction proliferated and health professionals assumed it was free of side effects or contraindications. Here is a case where medical practice benefits from study of the religious tradition, even as medical research helps to refine protections against religious "side effects."

---

[16] Gail Ironson et al., "The Ironson-Woods Spirituality/Religiousness Index Is Associated with Long Survival, Health Behaviors, Less Distress, and Low Cortisol in People with HIV/AIDS," *Annals of Behavioral Medicine* 24, no. 1 (2002): 34–48.
[17] Ingrid Provident and Kathleen Spadaro, *Health Benefits of Mindful Meditation*, ed. Jaime Uribarri and Joseph A. Vassalotti (Cham: Springer International Publishing, 2020).
[18] W. B. Britton et al., "Defining and Measuring Meditation-Related Adverse Effects in Mindfulness-Based Programs," *Clinical Psychological Science* 9, no. 6 (2021): 1185–204.
[19] See the Clinical and affective neuroscience laboratory at Brown. https://sites.brown.edu/britton/resources/.

Webs of Truth, Webs of Meaning

For a long time, the testimony of anecdotal experience and the traditions of clinical practice handed down within the medical community were not so different in kind from the testimony and traditions handed down in religious communities. Both put great weight on authority and texts, as well as observation and experience. The practice of medicine was perceived by those within and outside as having much in common with humanistic study more generally. But the methodologies have diverged.

In the medical sciences, truth is pursued through empirical data, with a sharp, exclusive focus on organic function. The data itself, what counts as evidence, is arranged in a hierarchy, a sort of pyramid. At the pinnacle, providing the supposed firmest evidence, stands the double-blinded, randomized, controlled trial. Below this level come other carefully designed observational or cohort studies, which follow and compare those receiving a treatment with a group that does not receive it, but without the prior randomization and blinding. At the lowest level stands clinical experience: reports from practitioners or clinics on the data in their immediate experience with a particular treatment. This hierarchy is complicated by a genre of meta-study that operates by collating other studies. This can be a systematic review, which simply collects and reports on the conclusions of all the studies relevant to a particular question. Or it can be a meta-analysis, which pools the raw information from many studies and makes them into one data base upon which the investigators perform their own statistical analysis.

The randomized controlled trial (RCT) is the most methodologically distinct of these approaches, and it holds a special pride of place in medical study. There are usually two study arms that are nearly identical as possible in all the characteristics of their constituent patients. One of the groups receives the target treatment, and the other receives an inactive simulation, a placebo.[20] Ideally, neither the patients in any group nor the health care professionals interacting directly with any participants know who belongs to which group. This is the "double blinding:" patients unaware of what they are receiving and health care professionals unaware of who belongs to what

---

[20]Or possibly, in a study with three "arms," there is a treatment group, a simulated treatment group (placebo), and a pure control group with no actual or apparent intervention.

group. Records are kept of both groups and at a stated interval, the data are "unblinded" and the outcomes for the treatment and the control groups compared.

To produce such "gold standard" evidence in medicine is expensive and labor-intensive. Even a small, short-term, RCT can cost millions of dollars. The design and interpretation of such studies require expertise—the work of clinicians, statisticians, research coordinators, and of course, patients—which is just as daunting to assemble as the money. Access to this kind of validation is thus extremely limited. Only a small percentage of potential therapies will ever have the opportunity for such testing. To these logistical difficulties have been added recent concerns about research fraud and a replication crisis.[21] When influential studies or experiments have been selected for replication, many have not had their results confirmed.[22] The many obstacles to performing high quality RCTs are multiplied for efforts at replication, not least in terms of ethical questions.[23] Since the best evidence requires both great expense and great expertise, and since much can ride on the results of a study (in terms of income for companies and institutions, as well as of promotion, security, and status for scholars), there can be implicit incentive to influence the outcome either through unconscious bias or outright fraud. An extremely influential paper on Alzheimer's disease was recently retracted, because it contained manipulated images and data.[24] This does not mean the thesis of the study itself was false, but the paper attracted many others to follow the same line of research on this devastating disease, and so may have wasted precious money, time, and opportunity.

The pyramid of evidence, so clear in theory, proves in fact to be more like a web. The relatively sparse, and often inconclusive data of RCTs is coordinated with observational studies and clinical experience. This is further complicated by the fact that much medical research is actually at

---

[21] David Hope, Avril Dewar, and Christopher Hay, "Is There a Replication Crisis in Medical Education Research?" *Academic Medicine* 96, no. 7 (2021): 958–63.

[22] Tara Haelle, "A Massive 8-Year Effort Finds That Much Cancer Research Cannot Be Replicated," *Science News,* December 7, 2021.

[23] If a medical RCT shows early evidence that the treatment group is gaining significant health benefits over the control group, ethical guidelines generally dictate that the blinding should be removed and the control group should now receive the treatment. Once it is clear that a benefit is being conferred, it is not fair to deny that benefit to those who were randomly excluded from it. But this raises the question of how one can deprive people of what has become a standard treatment in order to double check its original validation.

[24] Charles Piller, "Researchers Move to Retract Discredited Alzheimer's Study," *Science* 384, no. 6700 (2024): 1055.

several removes from testing actual outcomes in patients. These studies may experiment with the interactions of molecules, or test drug effects in animals, on a long path toward human trials. Medical practice remains an art, one that requires the ability to assimilate vast amounts of information in the face of uncertainty.

In contrast with the clarity of medicine's biological focus, the well-being sought by religion is wider and its evidence, though including effects on health, more diffuse. Religions too have their theoretical pyramids of evidence. Divine revelation and transcendent wisdom stand at the top, whether mediated through inspired texts, persons, or experiences. If the source is believed to be transcendent, the content can be given high evidentiary value. But revelation does not touch with equal relevance or clarity on all topics (including medical ones) and its interpretation required the application of other sources. Another type of evidence, thought to depend on or be grounded in revelation is the content of a religious tradition—its teachings, ritual practices, and communal authorities. Both of these sources are processed in the lives of individuals—intellectual, affective, and social. That is, their meaning is interpreted by means of rational reflection or argument as well as tested by experience.

Christian theology works through the correlation of these sources, the "quadrilateral" of scripture, tradition, reason, and experience. Each of these sources has its own practical internal hierarchy. Different Christian groups may give different parts of scripture higher effective authority than others, or prefer different philosophical traditions in applying reason, or prioritize different Christian confessional traditions, or emphasize different types of experience. Large areas of empirical agreement are still subject to evaluative divergence. For instance, we may agree that a given set of statements are all in scripture, but disagree on which of them should be the standard for interpreting the others.

The relation of reason and faith, of the empirical study prioritized in medicine and the self-transformational commitment involved in theology, has been a staple of theological reflection throughout Christian history. No single answer has probably been more influential than that of Thomas Aquinas, the preeminent thinker in the Roman Catholic tradition. For Aquinas, revelation gave access to truths that could not be known by reason, and reason gave access to information about the created world that had not been provided in revelation. Theology went beyond philosophy, but Aquinas argued that when both were done correctly they could not contradict each other. There was a relatively small area in which the two overlapped (something could be known by either philosophy or by revelation), and it was in this area that the two could be checked against each other.[25]

In the physical world, God normally works through secondary causes, which in medicine are biological and physiological processes. The empirical medicine just described is the study of such secondary causes, whose ultimate source is God. There is thus space for the exercise of independent medical reason. On the other hand, a theological perspective relativizes the purely medical understanding of human well-being within a wider one that includes relation with God and one's neighbors, which seeks not only physical health but moral regeneration, spiritual transformation, and a resurrected life beyond death. Health, meaning baseline effective organic function, is the aim and the standard for medicine. Transformation is the aim for religion, attainment of a spiritual, moral, and even physical condition that we have not previously known and cannot fully imagine.

This approach is far inferior to a biomedical one as directly applied to analysis of biological causality. But it has benefits in registering the evaluative and interpretive dimensions of health, and particularly in comprehending and correlating various types of truth. For instance, theology is used to thinking of its work as applying in a range of settings. There is theology that applies to worship and ritual, and theology that applies to community life and individual formation, theology that applies to service, as well as the theology we most often think of—intellectual understanding and interpretation.

The challenge for research in religion and health lies in coordinating these two very different approaches. The obstacles are both theoretical and practical. For instance, for ethical and practical reasons, a randomized control study is nearly impossible. People cannot be assigned to religious practice involuntarily or constrained from worship they would otherwise undertake. It would be impossible to "blind' such a study: people know if they are participating in religious activities or not, and whether their participation is genuine or feigned. Behavioral interventions (such as worship attendance) and attitudes (such as religiosity) do not come in the form of a pill or an isolated, distinct intervention and thus are extremely difficult to test.

---

[25] The existence of God and key elements of the moral law are examples of this. The existence of God should be knowable by sound reason, Aquinas argued, but it could also be believed simply on the basis of revelation.

The same factors that skew biomedical research apply to the study of religion and health. One of us heard a medical researcher investigating the uses of psychedelic drugs (such as psilocybin) to treat post-traumatic stress disorder complain about the difficulty in funding this work. The prospect that the drug might have a powerful long term effect based on only one or two applications—a very happy possibility from the point of view of patients' well-being—discouraged support from pharmaceutical companies that saw little prospect of consistent income from such a medication. Similarly, religious practices or participation cost the consumer nothing and so it is hard to find any to invest the resources required for high-quality studies to assess their effectiveness. Government agencies, the largest source of research funding, are hesitant to investigate therapies associated with religion.

It is all the more remarkable, then, that the sea change in research we discussed earlier in the chapter has taken place in the face of such difficulties. In the ten years from 2001 to 2010, the total number of studies almost tripled, from 1,200 to over 3,000.[26] A tabulation of all of these studies over nineteen different medical subject categories (such as suicide, depression, cholesterol, coronary disease, cancer, mortality) showed that positive associations of religion or spirituality with health vastly outnumbered negative associations in *every* category, by proportions of at least six to one.[27] Likening religious participation to a blockbuster drug (Lipitor) for only one medical condition, as we did at the start of this chapter, seems to far understate the case. It has the same dramatic relation with most conditions. This is the raw empirical data that places religion squarely in the medical realm.

Next Steps in Research

There is now not much debate over the positive associations of religion with health. The focus has shifted to how to interpret this data. Ironically, probably no topic illustrates the methodological issues better than the one that has often attracted the most public notice: studies on the medical effect of intercessory prayer. These studies fit the mold of modern religion-medicine research in that they are correlational. They are not focused on

---

[26]Koenig, "Religion, Spirituality, and Health: A Review and Update," 19.
[27]Ibid., 20.

miraculous medical outcomes in special cases, for none of the individual subjects in these studies claim to have experienced that. They focus instead on a statistical assessment of the correlation between remote prayer (which from a naturalistic perspective is not a causal variable at all) and specified medical outcomes. Publication in 1988 of a randomized control trial of intercessory prayer for cardiac patients, showing statistically significant positive variance for those prayed for, met with a "firestorm of comment and critique."[28] The critique came from the religiously skeptical and devout alike, and similar controversy has followed the periodic appearance of new studies of this sort, whatever their specific results.[29]

The sheer volume of research that has been done on this topic is surprising.[30] Some studies with positive results have been acknowledged, even by their critics to be methodologically sound. But this is less a proof of divine agency than a reminder that such trials, though a "gold standard" of research, can only register correlations and not mechanisms of action. This limitation is less evident when we can readily infer a plausible underlying causal path (the correlation makes intuitive sense) than it is when the implied path is not causal at according to normal medical understanding. The first lesson in any statistics class is, "Correlation does not imply causation."

The value of these prayer studies is greater in helping to clarify our methodological understanding of religion and medicine than it is in informing clinical practice. The studies raise the kind of questions we suggested earlier: how does one define and measure prayer? How could one have a true control group in such a study? Attempts to measure tangible medical effects of prayer run afoul of perhaps insurmountable difficulties in experimentally isolating its application and its recipients.[31] If groups are engaged to pray for some patients and not for others, there is no way to

---

[28]Jeffrey S. Levin, *Religion and Medicine: A History of the Encounter between Humanity's Two Greatest Institutions* (New York: Oxford University Press, 2020), 85.

[29]For instance, a large study in 2006 (also involving cardiac patients) indicated that those prayed for had *worse* outcomes than others. Herbert Benson et al., "Study of the Therapeutic Effects of Intercessory Prayer (Step) in Cardiac Bypass Patients: A Multicenter Randomized Trial of Uncertainty and Certainty of Receiving Intercessory Prayer," *The American Heart Journal* 151, no. 4 (2006): 934–42.

[30]See for instance the rigorous two volume review of such research on prayer and distance healing Daniel J. Benor, *Spiritual Healing: Scientific Validation of a Healing Revolution*, Healing Research (Southfield, MI: Vision Publications, 2001); *Spiritual Healing: Scientific Validation of a Healing Revolution: Professional Supplement*, Healing Research (Southfield, MI: Vision Publications, 2002).

[31]This is why we have explored the question of prayer in Chapter Four from a different perspective, seeing its effect as exercised in a modality that is not exclusive to prayer alone.

assure that the control group has not been the object of unknown prayer or simply the recipient of the generic prayers offered constantly by religious groups on behalf of "the sick."

The public attention given to these studies is unfortunate if it distracts attention from the extensive wider research literature we have been describing. These prayer studies are outliers precisely because the results have been so variable, while the research we have summarized is notable precisely for the consistent positive associations of religion and health. The prayer studies are outliers also in the sense that they appear to frustrate further inquiry, posing a blunt alternative: prayer works, or does not, by supernatural means inaccessible to rational understanding. The next steps in research in religion and health, on the other hand, involve a deeper exploration of what lies behind these positive associations.

Confounders

The relation between religion and health is complicated both by difficulties in defining and measuring religion and by versions of the same problems that bedevil all health research, particularly the difficulty in disentangling one factor's independent effect on health outcomes from all other factors. Once the correlation of religion and positive health outcomes become clear, the recurring objections to religion's significance do not deny the reality of the association, but deny that it is religion or faith specifically that is the active factor. Critics maintain that "religion" is standing in for something non-religious that comes along with religious practice, but has no necessary relation with it.

One criticism is that there may even be simple linguistic confusions. For example, in Ben's early research career, he studied the correlation of spirituality and depression in his medical practice.[32] He used validated questionnaires for depression and spiritually and asked his patients to fill them out. Sure enough, the more depressed patients were, the lower their spirituality scores. However, were not those two concepts really measuring the same thing? One item in the PHQ-9, a commonly used screening tool for

---

[32]Benjamin R. Doolittle and Michael Farrell, "The Association between Spirituality and Depression in an Urban Clinic," *Primary Care Companion to the Journal of Clinical Psychiatry* 6, no. 3 (2004): 114–18.

depression is, "Over the past 2 weeks, have you been down, depressed or hopeless."[33] An item from the widely used Spiritual Well-Being scale is, "I feel that life is full of conflict and unhappiness."[34] These items explore nearly the same domain, with slightly different wording. Surely, a person who feels depressed will also believe that life is filled with unhappiness. It is not surprising then that someone who scores highly on "purpose" would score lower on "hopelessness." Spirituality in these measures is not so much a distinct concept as it is a marker of general well-being. There are some elements of spirituality that are in truth distinctive, and can be differentiated, such as connection with the transcendent. But other aspects are more integral to positive mental health almost by definition, such as feeling a sense of purpose, recognizing goodness in the world.

Even well-designed research that finds a strong positive correlation between religious attendance or practice and health is subject to the critique that it may be indirectly measuring some other active variable. People who attend religious services are found to be healthier than those that do not. This could be the result of a selection bias. Only people of a certain level of health are capable of going to church, so in testing the health of church goers you have just preselected a population that will be healthier than a random group. Or perhaps religious attendance only indirectly affects health. There is another associated factor, not unique to religion, that explains the impact. Recently, researchers have highlighted the importance of social connection. Perhaps religious attendance builds social connections, and it is the social connections that improve health. Social connections produced by any means (bowling leagues, movie fan clubs) will perform equally well. From such a perspective, religious participation has an objective impact on health because it activates mediating causal agents, but these causes are not unique to religious activity.

Such "criticisms" have come a long way toward recognizing religion's positive effects on health. They are only arguing about how religious involvement produces those effects—through "secondary causes" or directly from some exclusively religious activity. We do not say a change in diet is not a true source for a health change because it is the changed glucose levels in

---

[33] Kurt Kroenke, Robert L. Spitzer, and Janet B. W. Williams, "The PHQ-9: Validity of a Brief Depression Severity Measure," *Journal of General Internal Medicine: JGIM* 16, no. 9 (2001): 432.

[34] Raymond F. Paloutzian et al., "The Spiritual Well-Being Scale (SWBS): Cross-Cultural Assessment across 5 Continents, 10 Languages, and 300 Studies," in *Assessing Spirituality in a Diverse World*, ed. Amy L. Ai, et al. (Cham: Springer International Publishing, 2021), 432.

the blood that are the proximate direct causes of changes in insulin production, and those glucose levels can also be changed by drugs, not just by diet.

However, research has recently become much more sophisticated in responding to these perennial objections, in teasing out the extent to which religious observance itself conveys a benefit, different from cooking classes and jogging clubs.[35] There is no better example than Tyler VanderWeele's work. VanderWeele is an epidemiologist and statistician of the first rank.[36] He and his co-authors published an article in 2016, based on the longitudinal data from the famous Framingham nurses study, which had assembled extensive medical and biographical information on a large cohort of Massachusetts nurses.[37] This data is publicly accessible, which means their findings can be verified by other scholars. The sample was large, including more than 70,000 participants. The researchers addressed the impracticality of a randomized controlled trial by studying participants over time, in this case over twelve years—a comparatively long time for such projects. They measured religious attendance at two different time-points as a proxy for consistency, breaking the categories for attendance into never, less than once a week, once a week, and more than once a week. The end points of the study were all cause mortality and mortality from heart disease and cancer. The bottom line conclusion was that weekly attendance at religious services reduced all-cause mortality by 33 percent.

Though notable for its size and rigor, the overall result of the study only replicated and confirmed what many others had found in terms of the correlation of religion and health. What stands out about VanderWeele's paper, the real headline, is the extent to which he used sophisticated statistical tools to painstakingly control for confounding variables. Virtually all the reasonable objections raised against other correlational studies are directly addressed. Perhaps religious attenders were simply healthier to begin with and sick people stay home. VanderWeele went through the data and controlled for baseline health status, so he could effectively say that among

---

[35] Tyler J. VanderWeele, "Religious Communities and Human Flourishing," *Current Directions in Psychological Science: A Journal of the American Psychological Society* 26, no. 5 (2017): 476–81.
[36] This is reflected in his Harvard professorship and his reception in 2017 of the President's Award from the Committee of Presidents of Statistical Societies, sometimes called the "Nobel Prize of statistics."
[37] Tyler VanderWeele et al., "Association of Religious Service Attendance with Mortality among Women," *Journal of the American Medical Association Internal Medicine* 176, no. 6 (2016): 777–85.

people with the same degree of heart disease, religious attenders still fared better than non-attenders. Perhaps the real reason for the improved longevity was social connections and friendships. He compared the religious with non-religious people with the same number of friends or social relations. The religious benefit remained. Perhaps mental health, or economic status, or ethnicity, or a personality trait like optimism, was the real determinant of the health outcomes and not attending worship. He controlled for those factors.

VanderWeele controlled for some twenty variables, from family income to access to medical care to diet, and came up with estimates as to how much of the positive health variance for religious attenders was accounted for by each one.[38] That is, the critics are correct that in some cases the confounding variables account for *some* portion of the variance. But the effect attributed only to the religious involvement remained distinct and robust.

Maybe there were variables that VanderWeele and his team simply did not consider. Musical taste? Political party? They tried to quantify the scale of this possibility as well. VanderWeele invented his own statistical test, the *E value*, which is used to answer the question, "If there was a variable we did not account for, some unmeasured influence, how large an effect would it need to be to negate the distinctive effect of religious observance?" He concluded that influence would have to have an effect more than twice as large as the total effect of all the other control variables combined.[39]

Such a study is a major step toward verifying that there is something actually religious at play in the relation of religion and health. It raises further fascinating questions. Religious attendance is a somewhat amorphous variable. What about this behavior is most significant in producing the observed effect? If it cannot be reduced to social cohesiveness, optimism, or something else, then what is it? VanderWeele performed a mediation analysis, which is a special statistic technique to associate underlying factors with the measured effect. Although religious observance has an effect above and beyond the features that were controlled for, it is associated with a constellation of these factors, a "set" that seems to hang together with religion, such as optimism and social integration, non-smoking, reduced alcohol consumption, and better diet quality. Whatever religion does "alone" it also seems to have an effect in drawing these various factors together. And

---

[38]See Table 1 in ibid., 780.
[39]ibid., 783.

after all, it is a strange definition of religion that *excludes* social connections or life style choices.

The data can tell us nothing about the motivation of these participants to attend worship. Do they attend out of joy and commitment to God, or from guilt and obligation, or something else? The snacks at coffee hour? In large, survey-based population studies, it is difficult to address questions about subjectivity. Due to the large, quantitative nature of VanderWeele's project, it cannot address what different perceptions of God or varied spiritual practices may exist within his population. That requires open-ended questions and qualitative analysis. The elegance of VanderWeele's project is that even this rather crude measure of religious participation—attendance—serves to highlight a real effect.

Of course further questions remain. This study dealt only with female nurses. Maybe there is something peculiar about nurses, unaddressed in VanderWeele's extensive statistical controls. However, similar studies have been performed in very different populations. A longitudinal study of people with HIV infection, a chronic disease, showed that monthly worship attendance reduced all-cause mortality by 10 percent. Although this is a modest reduction, the "dose" of religion was only once a month. Further analysis suggested that worship attendance was associated with fewer risk taking behaviors such as drug and alcohol use.[40]

The nurses' study was overwhelmingly composed of Catholic and Protestant Christians, and a small number of Jews. But the rubric for measuring religion, "religious service attendance," has no necessary limitation to those traditions. The medicine-faith conversation is inevitably an interfaith project. Indeed, the same correlation has been found for religious orientation in other faiths.[41] While the spiritual goods and aims of various traditions may be distinct, the correlatives to those aims in the sphere of health and well-being overlap to a very high degree. There are forms of asceticism, devotion, or service in all religious traditions that diverge from purely medical prescriptions for health or well-being. But each in some way also sees religious insight and commitment implicated in health.

---

[40] Benjamin R. Doolittle et al., "Mortality, Health, and Substance Abuse by Religious Attendance among HIV Infected Patients from the Veterans Aging Cohort Study," *AIDS and Behavior* 25, no. 3 (2021): 653–60.

[41] See for instance the study referred to above, which was cross-cultural and cross-religious. Hoogeveen et al., "A Many-Analysts Approach to the Relation between Religiosity and Well-Being."

Integration

Medicine seeks to isolate specific factors for health and tends towards reductionism. To cure disease, we seek the specific cell receptor to block, the exact gene to inhibit, the specific metabolic pathway to shut down. This is an important exercise because if we do not control for extraneous variables, we cannot trust the impact of our intervention.

There is a lab at Yale that explores how specific plant compounds impact health. For example, they extract molecules from kale and study how they might impact cancer cells. This is exciting work. But one learning might be just to eat more kale. There are likely many kale molecules that impact health, and they already come packaged in a perfect delivery vehicle, the cellulose matrix of the kale itself. The attempt to extract an essential ingredient may leave behind connections that make that ingredient effective. In the same way, we should not be reductionist when it comes to religion, since attempting to apply only one aspect of religious observance—social connection, for example—risks reducing its effect. Religious people may rightly ask why isolate specific features of religion? Just "eat more kale" by taking faith in its natural delivery package.

Religious traditions and communities come with holistic frameworks. They involve specific practices, but they commend them as part of an inclusive way of life. Research like VanderWeele's strongly supports the conclusion that there is an intrinsic health benefit in religion that is peculiarly religious. People of faith may call this grace, or forgiveness, or the work of the Holy Spirit. This does not deny that religious adherence also tends to integrate and mobilize many factors that are good for one's health in their own right.

People come together in community. Repeated studies show that social connection is a primary driver of well-being. Daniel Buettner has written extensively about all this in *The Blue Zones of Happiness: Lessons from the World's Happiest People*.[42] Those societies which foster strong social connection tend to have happier people and healthier people. Religious observance fosters social connection and community.

---

[42]Dan Buettner, *The Blue Zones of Happiness: Lessons from the World's Happiest People* (Washington, DC: National Geographic, 2017).

Religious observance engages intellectual activity. In most traditions, a religious leader will read sacred scripture and render a brief reflection on its relevance to life. In Christian traditions, this is the sermon; in Buddhism, the dharma talk; in Islam, the khutba. In a society where so many of us scroll needlessly through our social media apps, the sermon may be the most intellectual activity during the week, perhaps even more so than our professions.

Religious observance is artistic. In many traditions, we sing hymns. We chant. We contemplate the beautiful architecture of our worship spaces. In a society where we grind away at our jobs, numb ourselves in social media and cable television, religious observance gives us pause to consider beauty in the world, to *become* part of the creation of beauty.

Religious observance reorients us to the transcendent, to God. We pray. We examine ourselves from a vantage point that relativizes us, not from the usual one that relativizes everything by reference to us. We seek forgiveness and reconciliation. We petition our hopes. This reorients us to others and quickens us to virtue and meaning. Finally, religious beliefs constitute an ultimate horizon for our lives, one whose meaning can uphold us even in the face of defeats and trials.

Part of religion's effect on health is a motivational and integrative one. There are elements that can improve our health, but we need a reason to actualize them. The challenge with mindfulness is that we download the Calm app but never use it. We consider building relationships, but then reach for our phones. Faith engages the mysterious, seamless unity of a way of life that is constantly remaking us. It reflects the paradox of something that is good for us in many respects precisely because it animates us to care about something beyond ourselves. This explains the hesitancy of many religious people to approach religion in a scientifically experimental way, in the conviction that the religion defined by such study will be a shell of what religion actually is. To treat religion as if it is always about what is in our interest:—improving our health, serving our selfish well-being—tends to ignore if not to undermine what actually gives it that kind of therapeutic power.

We can end this chapter on evidence on religion and health by noting that there is even research that bears on the specific topic of this book: the importance of a harmonious relation between religion and medicine. The investigators took as their point of departure the large body of evidence that "suggests people who hold religious/spiritual (R/S) beliefs tend to experience higher levels of well-being (i.e., physical and mental health) than people who lack such beliefs."[43] All things being equal, religious beliefs correspond with better health outcomes. The authors note that there is a smaller, but growing body of research that indicates the same is true for people who hold positive attitudes toward science (a positive attitude meaning that whatever the state of their knowledge of scientific content, they have an accepting outlook toward science). Positive views toward science also correlate with well-being.

They then took a logical step beyond these two data points to investigate the value of people's experienced *consonance* between their religious and scientific attitudes. As one might intuitively suspect, the investigators found that such consonance itself correlated with higher levels of well-being. Their results suggest that a harmonious or mutually supportive orientation toward science and religion tends to maximize the positive health benefits of each attitude individually. A perceived conflict or hostility between the two, to some extent, diminishes the health benefits correlated with both.

This study focuses on science generally, but we can suppose that it applies equally to medicine as a subset of science. The authors note that the health benefits of pro-religious and pro-scientific outlooks are best attested in Western societies (where the largest number of studies have been done). It is also true that the conflict between religion and science, which shadows the interactions of medicine and faith, is not a cultural constant. It has existed in its most acute form only in the modern west, making our societies rather odd in global perspective.[44] The authors conclude that, in this light, the perceived incompatibility between religious/spiritual and pro-science belief systems becomes "not just a matter of academic or cultural debate, but an issue with important repercussions for psychological well-being and, therefore, public health."[45] A tendency for religious and scientific-medical perspectives to interfere with each other is, perhaps, a malady more widespread in our cultures than in many others. And conversations like that in this book are part of its diagnosis and treatment.

---

[43] Michael E. Price and Dominic D. P. Johnson, "Science and Religion Around the World: Compatibility between Belief Systems Predicts Increased Well-Being," *Religion, Brain & Behavior* (2024): 1, https://doi.org/10.1080/2153599X.2024.2363773. The following paragraphs summarize the content of this article.

[44] See for instance Elaine Howard Ecklund et al., *Secularity and Science: What Scientists around the World Really Think About Religion* (Oxford University Press, 2019), doi:10.1093/oso/9780190926755.001.0001.

[45] Price and Johnson, "Science and Religion around the World: Compatibility between Belief Systems Predicts Increased Well-Being," 16.

References

Benor, Daniel J. *Spiritual Healing: Scientific Validation of a Healing Revolution.* Healing Research. Southfield, MI: Vision Publications, 2001.

Benor, Daniel J. *Spiritual Healing: Scientific Validation of a Healing Revolution: Professional Supplement.* Healing Research. Southfield, MI: Vision Publications, 2002.

Benson, Herbert, Jeffery A. Dusek, Jane B. Sherwood, Peter Lam, Charles F. Bethea, William Carpenter, Sidney Levitsky, et al. "Study of the Therapeutic Effects of Intercessory Prayer (Step) in Cardiac Bypass Patients: A Multicenter Randomized Trial of Uncertainty and Certainty of Receiving Intercessory Prayer." [In English]. *The American Heart Journal* 151, no. 4 (2006): 934–42.

Britton, W.B., J.R. Lindahl, D.J. Cooper, N.K. Canby, and R. Palitsky. "Defining and Measuring Meditation-Related Adverse Effects in Mindfulness-Based Programs." [In English]. *Clinical Psychological Science* 9, no. 6 (2021): 1185–204.

Buettner, Dan. *The Blue Zones of Happiness: Lessons from the World's Happiest People.* Washington, DC: National Geographic, 2017.

Deikman, Arthur J. "Review of Mysticism: Spiritual Quest or Psychic Disorder?" *Journal of Nervous and Mental Disease* 165 (1977): 214.

Doolittle, Benjamin R., Kathleen McGinnis, Yusuf Ransome, David Fiellin, and Amy Justice. "Mortality, Health, and Substance Abuse by Religious Attendance among HIV Infected Patients from the Veterans Aging Cohort Study." [In English]. *AIDS and Behavior* 25, no. 3 (2021): 653–60.

Doolittle, Benjamin R., and Michael Farrell. "The Association between Spirituality and Depression in an Urban Clinic." [In English]. *Primary Care Companion to the Journal of Clinical Psychiatry* 6, no. 3 (2004): 114–18.

Ecklund, Elaine Howard, David R. Johnson, Brandon Vaidyanathan, Kirstin R.W. Matthews, Steven W. Lewis, Robert A. Thomson, and Di Di. *Secularity and Science: What Scientists Around the World Really Think About Religion.* Oxford University Press, 2019. doi:10.1093/oso/9780190926755.001.0001.

Haelle, Tara. "A Massive 8-Year Effort Finds That Much Cancer Research Cannot Be Replicated." *Science News,* December 7, 2021.

Hall, Daniel E. "Religious Attendance: More Cost-Effective Than Lipitor?" [In English]. *Journal of the American Board of Family Medicine* 19, no. 2 (2006): 103–9.

Hoogeveen, Suzanne, Alexandra Sarafoglou, Balazs Aczel, Yonathan Aditya, Alexandra J. Alayan, Peter J. Allen, Sacha Altay, et al. "A Many-Analysts Approach to the Relation between Religiosity and Well-Being." [In English]. *Religion, Brain & Behavior* 13, no. 3 (2023): 237–83.

Hope, David, Avril Dewar, and Christopher Hay. "Is There a Replication Crisis in Medical Education Research?" [In English]. *Academic Medicine* 96, no. 7 (2021): 958–63.

Ironson, Gail, George F. Solomon, Elizabeth G. Balbin, Conall O'Cleirigh, Annie George, Mahendra Kumar, David Larson, and Teresa E. Woods. "The Ironson-Woods Spirituality/Religiousness Index Is Associated with Long Survival, Health Behaviors, Less Distress, and Low Cortisol in People with HIV/Aids." [In English]. *Annals of behavioral medicine* 24, no. 1 (2002): 34–48.

Koenig, Harold G., Dana E. King, and Verna Benner Carson. *Handbook of Religion and Health*. 2nd ed. Oxford; New York: Oxford University Press, 2012.

Koenig, Harold G.M.D. "Religion, Spirituality, and Health: A Review and Update." *Advances in Mind—Body Medicine* 29, no. 3 (2015): 19–26.

Kroenke, Kurt, Robert L. Spitzer, and Janet B. W. Williams. "The Phq-9: Validity of a Brief Depression Severity Measure." [In English]. *Journal of General Internal Medicine: JGIM* 16, no. 9 (2001): 606–13.

Larson, David B., and Susan S. Larson. *The Forgotten Factor in Physical and Mental Health: What Does the Research Show?: An Independent Study Seminar*. Rockville, MD: National Institute for Healthcare, 1994.

Larson, David B., Jeffrey S. Levin, and Harold G. Koenig. *Faith, Medicine, and Science: A Festschrift in Honor of Dr. David B. Larson*. Binghamton, NY: Haworth Pastoral Press, 2005.

Larson, Susan S. "David: My Daring, Dauntless, Devoted White Knight." In *Faith, Medicine, and Science: A Festschrift in Honor of Dr. David B. Larson*, edited by David B. Larson, Jeffrey S. Levin, and Harold G. Koenig, xxvi, 321p. Binghamton, NY: Haworth Pastoral Press, 2005.

Levin, Jeffrey S. *Religion and Medicine: A History of the Encounter between Humanity's Two Greatest Institutions*. New York: Oxford University Press, 2020.

Osler, William. "The Faith That Heals." [In English]. *BMJ (Online)* 1, no. 2581 (1910): 1470–2.

Paloutzian, Raymond F., Zuhâl Agilkaya-Sahin, Kay C. Bruce, Marianne Nilsen Kvande, Klara Malinakova, Luciana Fernandes Marques, Ahmad S. Musa, et al. "The Spiritual Well-Being Scale (Swbs): Cross-Cultural Assessment across 5 Continents, 10 Languages, and 300 Studies." In *Assessing Spirituality in a Diverse World*, edited by Amy L. Ai, Paul Wink, Raymond F. Paloutzian and Kevin A. Harris, 413–44. Cham: Springer International Publishing, 2021.

Piller, Charles. "Researchers Move to Retract Discredited Alzheimer's Study." *Science* 384, no. 6700 (2024): 1055.

Price, Michael E., and Dominic D.P. Johnson. "Science and Religion around the World: Compatibility between Belief Systems Predicts Increased Well-Being." *Religion, Brain & Behavior* (2024): 1–20. https://doi.org/10.1080/2153599X.2024.2363773.

Provident, Ingrid, and Kathleen Spadaro. *Health Benefits of Mindful Meditation.* Edited by Jaime Uribarri and Joseph A. Vassalotti, 159–76. Cham: Springer International Publishing, 2020.

Rosmarin, David H., and Harold G. Koenig. *Handbook of Spirituality, Religion, and Mental Health.* 2nd ed. London; San Diego, CA: Academic Press, an imprint of Elsevier, 2020.

Schweninger, Loren. "Counting the Costs: Southern Planters and the Problem of Runaway Slaves, 1790–1860." [In English]. *Business and Economic History* 28, no. 2 (1999): 267–75.

VanderWeele, Tyler J. "Religious Communities and Human Flourishing." [In English]. *Current Directions in Psychological Science: A Journal of the American Psychological Society* 26, no. 5 (2017): 476–81.

VanderWeele, Tyler J., Li Sharshan, Meir J. Stampfar, and David R. Williams. "Association of Religious Service Attendance with Mortality among Women." *Journal of the American Medical Association Internal Medicine* 176, no. 6 (2016): 777–85.

7

Faith and Contagion in the Public Square

Chapter Outline

Contagion Changes Everything	132
Plague and Religion	135
Disease and Disgust	139
The Scapegoat Prescription	141
Relevance of the Past	145

A terrible infection afflicts countries around the world. Cities establish field hospitals in open lots. Schools, offices, factories, and religious institutions shut down. Many flee their homes to distant places they hope will be safer. Millions die. Readers can readily recognize these images from their own experience of the Covid-19 pandemic. That pandemic introduced new generations to a lethal reality all too common throughout history.[1]

This chapter offers us a different perspective on our topic of medicine and religion in two respects. First, it illustrates the importance of this connection in our analytical understanding of the past—not only the histories of medicine and of religion but the history of our societies as a whole. Medical

---

[1] Teaching our class online during the pandemic was a humbling experience, as each week members checked in from their different vantage points: Ben from the wards of Yale New Haven Hospital treating Covid-19 patients, one student from her role as a city public health officer, another as a minister to dying patients, another from a locked down apartment shared with elderly at-risk parents. All this encouraged us to look anew at this dimension of our topic.

crises have often affected the course of religious movements and, conversely, religious orientations have often shaped cultural and social responses to such medical challenges. This is not simply an antiquarian interest. Such examples suggest to us how this process continues to play out in our own time. Second, this chapter turns our focus away from individual bedsides to a context in which it is society itself that is the patient. Death and disease typically appear entirely as incidents in personal stories. But at times they are a shared social experience, one with its own peculiar medical and religious dimensions.

Contagion Changes Everything

Medicine is practiced in intensively individual terms. Contagious diseases, especially those with high mortality rates, add an unavoidable social dimension to this picture. Covid, smallpox, and HIV are suffered by individuals, but they are contracted through interaction with others. Depending on the infection, the necessary interaction could range from intimate bodily contact to breathing the air in the same vicinity. Everyone, infected or not, experiences secondary symptoms of a pandemic—isolation, anxiety, economic loss. Those symptoms are mediated through our web of human relationships and through the social actions taken to support public health. Normal human relations become vectors of possible harm, and the disease thus afflicts our families, our employment, our recreations.

Societies can be said to suffer from the sicknesses of individuals, for example in the cumulative years of life and productivity lost to heart disease or cancer. But the toll of epidemics is immediate. As symptoms of epidemics are experienced beyond the bodies of those directly infected, so epidemics call forth "treatments" that are society-wide and that exceed what we would usually consider medical. Here is a reminder that many of the gains we attribute to modern medicine come not from cures but from prevention, from changes at the community level in sanitation, nutrition, and shelter. This is famously illustrated in John Snow's isolation of the source of an 1854 cholera epidemic in London to a single water pump.[2] Dramatic declines

---

[2] Narushige Shiode et al., "The Mortality Rates and the Space-Time Patterns of John Snow's Cholera Epidemic Map," *International Journal of Health Geographics* 14, no. 1 (2015): 21.

in cholera deaths were driven by social systems for the disposal of waste and provision of clean water, more than treatment modalities. A similar thing can be said of the high proportion of maternal deaths from "childbed fever" that an Austrian doctor discovered to be caused by infection carried on the hands of attending physicians: the "cure" was regularized hand washing.[3]

One death or debilitating sickness can devastate and reconstitute a family. An epidemic is a sickness of an entire community. At the extreme, it can unravel and reorder a society, not only killing a percentage of the population but altering social norms, economic and political systems, and religions. Initially, epidemics can call forth a solidarity across the usual social divisions, prompted by a common threat, much as people may come together in times of war. People feel their common humanity and their common vulnerability in a new way. Indeed, medieval artistic representations of the plague tend to express a macabre satisfaction in its leveling effects, as the disease carries off the rich and the powerful with no regard for their privilege. But the main distinction of major contagious diseases is that they can change the health and viability of entire communities. In a pandemic, an affliction visits the entire society and compels a response that affects all parts of it.

William McNeill's 1976 book *Plagues and Peoples* reminded modern readers, grown indifferent to the constancy of epidemics in history, of the scope of their importance.[4] He pointed out contagious disease was often a major factor at turning points in world history, though rarely acknowledged as such by historians. The advent of the African slave trade in North America was catalyzed by measles and smallpox, viruses that killed nearly 98 percent of the local population in Hispaniola when Spanish adventurers invaded there in the 1400s. That devastation allowed a handful of conquistadores to conquer the island, but also depleted the population from which they sought slave labor. Since the indigenous populations were so diminished, the conquistadores began importing Africans to mine and to cultivate sugar cane, begetting a centuries long oppression whose legacy surrounds us now. Slavery, in turn, spawned a medical specialization that defined health in

---

[3] See Nicholas Kadar, Roberto Romero, and Zoltán Papp, "Ignaz Semmelweis: The 'Savior of Mothers': On the 200th Anniversary of His Birth," *American Journal of Obstetrics and Gynecology* 219, no. 6 (2018): 519–22.
[4] William Hardy McNeill, *Plagues and Peoples*, 1st ed. (Garden City, NY: Anchor Press, 1976).

terms of the value of human property and that promulgated racist assumptions on the physiology of African Americans.[5]

Napoleon's famous invasion of Russia looms large in European history, but contagious disease decided its outcome more than any general or battle. When it crossed the Niemen River into Russia in June 1812, Napoleon's Grand Armée numbered nearly half a million soldiers. As he approached Moscow, an outbreak of dysentery killed 120,000, vastly overshadowing the effects of the only major battle of the entire invasion—the Battle of Borodino—which resulted in 30,000 French casualties. As Napoleon fled Russia, an outbreak of typhus and other infectious diseases decimated the remainder of his army. By November, five months after invading, only 10,000 soldiers survived to cross the border towards France. The vast majority had died of infectious disease as well as frigid temperatures and starvation.[6] Subtract contagious disease from this picture, and the map of Europe would look vastly different.

Every pandemic is also a kind of diagnostic scan of a society, revealing comorbidities that exacerbate its effects. Some of these may be circumstantial: tightly packed urban populations fare worse than those sprinkled over a rural landscape. Others may reflect inequities magnified by disease. Those with better access to health care have better outcomes than those without it. For instance, a Harvard study among Covid-19 patients in Massachusetts showed that mortality was 40 percent higher in cities and towns with the largest minority concentration. Mortality was 14 percent higher in the most crowded cities compared with the least, and 9 percent higher in those with the worst poverty.[7]

The poor and disenfranchised tend to suffer more than others when pandemics hit, whether in fifth-century BCE Athens, fourteenth-century Florence, or twenty-first-century New York, Arizona, or Texas. In fact, this may be more true today than it was in medieval times, when medical care

---

[5] See for instance, Chapter One in Carolyn Roberts' groundbreaking dissertation, Carolyn Roberts, *To Heal and to Harm: Medicine, Knowledge, and Power in the Atlantic Slave Trade* (Cambridge, MA: Harvard University Press, 2017). See also Todd L. Savitt, "Black Health on the Plantation: Owners, the Enslaved, and Physicians," *OAH Magazine of History* 19, no. 5 (2005): 14–16.

[6] See Chapter Nine, War and Disease: Napoleon, Dysentery, and Typhus in Russia, 1812, in Frank M. Snowden, *Epidemics and Society: From the Black Death to the Present*, The Open Yale Courses Series (New Haven, CT: Yale University Press, 2019).

[7] Nancy Krieger, Pamela D. Waterman, and Jarvis T. Chen, "Covid-19 and Overall Mortality Inequities in the Surge in Death Rates by Zip Code Characteristics: Massachusetts, January 1 to May 19, 2020," *American Journal of Public Health* 110, no. 12 (2020): 1850–2.

could make less of a difference. Pandemics show up existing cracks in our society and may create new ones, whether these run between those who can work at home and those who must work in contact with others, or between those who can afford new treatments and those that cannot. The response to a contagious disease affects the entire texture of society, and so it will involve decisions by governments and institutions on resource allocation and on rules and guidance.

Plague and Religion

In European history and imagination, one pattern for contagious disease stands out above others. In 1347, a ship from the Black Sea sailed into the Sicilian port of Messina. On board were flea-infested rats carrying *Yersinia pestis*. Over the next few years, 30–50 percent of the population of Western Europe died of the bubonic plague. This was but the regional face of a global epidemic disease truly unusual both in the high mortality rate of those affected and in the short, violent course of their demise.[8] This cataclysmic upheaval was repeated again in the fifteenth century. The sum effect of the disease, starting with the decline in population, affected everything in society, from the labor supply to art. The subsequent transformations of Europe, including the Reformation and the Renaissance and the rise of city states and the mercantile class, all grew in social soil ravaged by plague.[9]

Pandemics have affected religion just as they affected every other aspect of society. This was particularly so since religion was itself the prime frame within which victims and survivors interpreted the event. When Attila the Hun and his armies arrived at Rome in 452, he met with Pope Leo and subsequently decided to withdraw rather than attacking the city. This retreat was subsequently attributed to the Pope's intervention or to divine power. But plague had been ravaging northern Italy and its appearance among Attila's soldiers was a concrete incentive for his withdrawal. The legendary accounts reflect the ease with which the medical and the religious perspectives on epidemics have intermingled. The modern distinction between plague and divine intervention was foreign at the time and to many subsequent

---

[8]See Chapter Three in Snowden, *Epidemics and Society: From the Black Death to the Present*.
[9]See Faye Marie Getz, "Black Death and the Silver Lining: Meaning, Continuity, and Revolutionary Change in Histories of Medieval Plague," *Journal of the History of Biology* 24, no. 2 (1991): 265–89.

historians: plague *was* divine intervention. It might be sent to punish offenders, chastise and purify believers, or guide the path of history. Plague, after all, had been among the instruments God used to free the people of Israel from their bondage in slavery. As the natural mechanisms of its operation were mysterious and seemingly arbitrary, the scope for religious interpretation was vast.

Plague clearly shaped the practice of faith. We saw in Chapter Five that the epidemic breakdown of society left people without priests to pastor the dying. The result was the proliferation of the *ars moriendi* texts, popular "do it yourself" guides for self-examination and preparation for death. The church emerged from this period weakened by the loss of a large proportion of its leaders and marked by more tension between clergy and laity.[10] The plague centuries also saw the development of radical and populist religious movements, such as the flagellants who practiced severe self mortification as a form of repentance in face of the disease. This ferment fueled the rise of reform movements that culminated in the Reformation. We saw in Chapter 3, with the example of the Isenheim altarpiece, how Christian devotion could tune its imagery to specific medical conditions. In the wake of the plague, the physical images of Christ and of Mary were transformed in art. The body of Christ on the cross grows more anguished and bloody, Mary's grief is frequently represented, with palpable emotion. The images of martyrs persevering through death become more realistic. All of these themes loom larger in imagination and devotion. Some of what later moderns regard as lurid tones in this imagery borrowed from the literal reality of that time.

Epidemics threatened the basic function of social institutions. They strained even intimate ties among family members when care carried the dangers of contagion. And epidemics challenged people's fundamental sense of meaning. Plague sows political and religious doubt as well as physical disease. Faith in divine providence and goodness falters in the face of such catastrophe, but then so does investment in the secular goods that might substitute for it: romance, cultural achievement, financial or political power.

As epidemics shaped religious history, so religious responses to epidemics have shaped history as well. We can consider the role of plague in the rise of Christianity. The early centuries of the common era saw two major epidemic waves in the Roman world, the Antonine plague (165–180 BCE) and the

---

[10] Alexander Clarence Flick, *The Decline of the Medieval Church*, Burt Franklin Bibliography & Reference Series, (New York: B. Franklin, 1967), 337.

plagues of Cyprian (250–270 BCE). Historians are well acquainted with the observations by early Christian writers who claimed that Christians stood out from their neighbors for the level of their mutual care, and even for their care of those outside the church during these epidemics. Scholars have generally discounted these as triumphal apologies for the church.

But sociologist Rodney Stark recently revisited this question through the lens of public health and suggested that the Christian response might well have been a key element in the growth of the church.[11] Of course, the social upheaval that comes with mass death scrambles society and opens space for new developments. It is often remarked that religious "revitalization movements" are common in such settings, as for instance among Native Americans in the wake of European colonialism. Certain features of Christianity's beliefs and practices may have situated it to negotiate the epidemics in an incrementally different manner than other communities, one whose ultimate effect was to grow Christians as a proportion of that society.

The key medical point Stark raises is expressed in a quote from McNeill: "When all normal services break down, quite elementary nursing will greatly reduce mortality."[12] People who would otherwise die, because they become too weak to obtain basic necessities on their own, may survive if given only the support that friends or family normally provide. Stark's medical estimates suggest such care could cut mortality rates significantly, as much as a half to two thirds. Even when the remaining mortality rate was still horrific, this is a dramatic difference. Stark argues that the behavior attributed to Christians—they stayed by their afflicted family and community members, accepting the risk to themselves—would translate into providing this care in greater proportion than other groups, and so lead to lower mortality and a greater number of survivors.

As to why Christians would do this, Stark points to prior beliefs and practices, ones not created by the plague, but evident in response to it. Christians were more hopeful of a future life, and so more ready to bear the risk of caring for the sick. Their communities organized to function as

---

[11] For what follows in this paragraph and the next two, see Chapter Four, "Epidemics, Networks, and Conversion," in Rodney Stark, *The Rise of Christianity: How the Obscure, Marginal Jesus Movement Became the Dominant Religious Force in the Western World in a Few Centuries*, 1st HarperCollins pbk. ed. (San Francisco, CA: HarperSanFrancisco, 1997).
[12] Ibid., 88.

miniature welfare states, providing care to each other.[13] Christians viewed those who gave their lives in care for the sick as admirable, akin to martyrs, emulating their Lord. They already had adopted mutual aid and care as a key expectation and practice within their communities. By contrast, Galen, the revered model physician, lived in Rome during the first of these plague periods. He left Rome for Asia Minor, to get out of harm's way.[14] There was nothing unusual or irrational about that behavior: it requires a distinctive kind of community to produce a contrary expectation.

In a famous letter in 362 CE, the Emperor Julian, who sought to reinstate traditional Roman religions and resist Christianity, wrote (unhappily) to one of his priests, "For when none of the Jews beg, and the impious Galileans relieve both their own poor and ours it is shameful that ours should be destitute of our assistance."[15] The relative neglect of the pagan poor was so evident to Julian that he argued "the impious Galileans observed this fact and devoted themselves to philanthropy" as a kind of competitive strategy.[16]

Stark argues that to the extent Christians extended their care to those beyond the church, they improved the differential survival of those who would prove most likely to subsequently join the church, either in gratitude or because Christian social networks had replaced their previous ones. Stark (in agreement with most other historians) estimates that early Christianity grew from well less than 1 percent of the population prior to the plague of 165 to 2 percent prior to the plague of 251, and then rapidly to upwards of 10 percent in the wake of the 252 plague, and finally to more than 50 percent by 350. He differs from his colleagues in regarding the plagues as a major factor, more significant, for instance, than Constantine's adoption of Christianity. That conversion came at the very end of the process Stark describes, and would not have happened had Christianity not already grown to this extraordinary extent. A differential religious response to the waves of disease played a key role in the transformation of the Roman Empire.

---

[13] The term comes from Paul Johnson, *A History of Christianity*, 1st American ed. (New York: Atheneum, 1976). 75.
[14] Stark, *The Rise of Christianity: How the Obscure, Marginal Jesus Movement Became the Dominant Religious Force in the Western World in a Few Centuries*, 85–6.
[15] David Ayerst and A.S.T. Fisher, *Records of Christianity*, 2 vols., vol. 1 (Oxford: B. Blackwell, 1971), 179.
[16] Ibid., 181.

Disease and Disgust

We saw in Chapter Four that our bodies are not passive subjects of pain and disease. There are internal biological processes that intensify or inhibit our experience of pain. There are the proactive defense mechanisms of our immune system that defend, heal, and, at times, attack us. There are explicit and implicit frameworks of meaning and belief that affect health outcomes. All of this exists, analogously, on a social level. Our social immune system, for instance, involves structures such as sewage systems and food inspection regulations, and our medical institutions, all of which maintain health at the population level. Our religious/cultural immune system involves the structures of meaning and common value that undergird the social immune system and guide our response to new challenges, like epidemics.

Religious and medical perspectives overlap at a profound psychological level. This is evident in typical human responses of revulsion and disgust. These vary slightly in cultural detail, but all people feel a level of disgust and avoidance in respect to what is expelled from our bodies (feces, urine, vomit, blood) and in respect to what has the smell or consistency of rotten food. There is a good biological basis for this response. Contact with bodily fluids can transmit disease and ingesting spoiled food is also dangerous. An intuitive avoidance of contamination is part of well-being.

These categories—purity, disgust—are culturally expanded to apply to things regarded as morally or spiritually unhealthy: incest, torture of animals, physical abuse of one person (especially a weaker one) by another. Every religion has incorporated imagery and emotions related to purity: dietary codes, rituals of purification, special spaces and times that are not to be profaned with certain kinds of behavior. The biological revulsion that we feel over contact with certain physical objects is transferred to the moral and spiritual realm. For instance, in experiments, most people refuse to put on a sweater that they are told was worn by Hitler.[17] Though we know that evil is not transmitted the way a virus is, we tend to treat the two in the same psychological register.

We can see then why contagious disease has a special place in the interface of religion and medicine. Concern for contagion and contamination is

---

[17] Richard Allan Beck, *Unclean: Meditations on Purity, Hospitality, and Morality* (Eugene, OR.: Cascade Books, 2011), 25–6.

deeply wired in us, and it is not intuitively easy for us to isolate the physical from the spiritual. We may say that only ancient superstition treated the ill as "unclean," but it is not unusual to treat someone as contaminated in a social or relational sense. Many cancer patients, for example, report sensing a kind of revulsion/avoidance from those around them, as though the condition could be caught.[18] Contagious disease and moral or spiritual contamination run together, with important effects in both medicine and religion.

This is why literature regularly turns to plague as an image for our ultimate existential state. The theme runs from Sophocles' *Oedipus* through Camus' *The Plague*. Oedipus' discovery of his marriage to his mother and murder of his father results from his quest as king of Thebes to find the cause of the disease that afflicted the city. As king-priest-physician, it is his task to uncover and remedy the cause of the plague, a source commonly expected to take the form of some deep and shocking moral or ritual transgression. When a sickness afflicts the entire community, it falls to those in authority for the whole community to find the treatment (which in this case is the ostracization and punishment of Oedipus) that accords with the intelligibility of the illness (its source in a moral offense). The lack of a remedy or an explanation multiplies the devastation, undermining not only bodily health but social and metaphysical confidence.

In Camus' account of the plague's mysterious arrival in a North African city, he incorporates all these prior religious and cultural dimensions. While they remain vital in their own right—his characters have genuine religious and medical struggles—these factors become a parable for European life under another kind of infection, the Nazi occupation. The existential crises prompted by epidemics seem to Camus to mirror those raised by living in a web of complicity with inhuman oppression. Epidemics prompt existential crises: religious doubts over the plague's meaning, social doubts about commitment to disintegrating institutions and norms, tensions between concern for one's own life and commitments to neighbor. These are the same crises, Camus suggests, that arise when the spreading sickness is ideological and moral.

The religious dimension of pandemics is not limited to consideration of God as their proximate cause—the God-virus connection, we might say. It is even more at issue in our relations with each other under the threat of

---

[18]See C. Vrinten et al., "Cancer Stigma and Cancer Screening Attendance: A Population-Based Survey in England," *BMC Cancer* 19, no. 1 (2019): 566.

epidemics. What we know to be an impersonal biological process is yet transmuted into behavior that has a decidedly moralistic frame. The Covid epidemic gave us a vivid glimpse of this dynamic. People whose health status might pose a threat to my own can readily be believed to be willfully or purposely culpable for that threat. When a co-worker got a Covid-19 infection, we wondered if they were vaccinated or if they were wearing a mask.

The Scapegoat Prescription

One long-standing religious diagnosis and prescription for pandemics is as relevant as it ever was. It is a treatment applied in the face of social crisis, and pandemics are a paradigm case of such crisis. To illustrate this, consider another historical case. In 430 BCE, a pandemic afflicted the Greek-speaking world, Athens in particular. Evidence suggests that the infection was a form of typhus, but other compelling candidates include typhoid and measles.[19] Thucydides, the Athenian historian who gave eyewitness account of the plague, wrote, "The disease began with a strong fever in the head and reddening and burning in the eyes; the first internal symptoms were that the throat and tongue became bloody and the breath unnatural and malodorous . . . Most victims then suffered from empty retching, which induced violent convulsion . . . Most died about the seventh or the ninth day."[20] Anywhere from 25–50 percent of the population perished, including leaders like Pericles, Athens' leading politician, and key figures in all phases of community life. In wake of the disease, government crumbled and the democratic institutions of the time gave way to more autocratic forms. Many forms of religious practice were abandoned, and temples left unattended. There was a collapse of social norms. People raided homes of the dead, committed acts of violence against each other, and turned their backs even on their own family members. Geo-political consequences followed, as Athens lost the second Peloponnesian War to Sparta, ending their regional dominance for generations.

---

[19] Burke A. Cunha, *The Cause of the Plague of Athens: Plague, Typhoid, Typhus, Smallpox, or Measles?* (Philadelphia: Elsevier Inc, 2004).
[20] Thucydides, *The Peloponnesian War* (Cambridge: Hackett 1998), 98.

The description just given left out an important feature in the Athenian response to the plague. The city employed an ancient practice that was already validated both by religion and custom.[21] Athens maintained an imprisoned cohort of criminals and captives for the performance of a particular ritual in response to threats to the community, particularly one like the plague. The imprisoned individuals were driven through the streets, with the whole city turning out to beat and abuse them. They might, at different times in Athen's history, have been forced to jump off a cliff or stoned. The end point for these battered victims was either death by collective execution or physical expulsion, with the expectation this ritual violence would bring an end to the epidemic or ameliorate its effect.

The word used to denote the persons sacrificed in this way was *pharmakos*, from which we get our word pharmacy. The word could mean either poison or cure (reflecting the belief that a remedy might often be a modulated dose of the cause). In fact, such victims were identified with the cause of the epidemic and their elimination with the remedy for it. Though the Athenians knew nothing of microbes, we could say the *pharmakoi* were treated as the contamination in the body and their elimination as the treatment for the disease. Striking out against them as one would at the cause of the epidemic or the epidemic itself was a cathartic and unifying social action. Scapegoating, in other words, is an ancient therapeutic prescription for epidemics.[22]

To historians, this Athenian practice is an odd footnote to the plague story. But it is not peculiar to this case. It is repeated across cultures and time periods.[23] Plainly, such rituals had no effect on the behavior of germs or viruses. However, they focused the felt need for a culprit, someone to blame, and they united the community (or tried to) in the midst of the dissolving social norms and mutual suspicion that mass disease produces. Such religious activity may not have blocked viral contagion in individual bodies: it did in fact treat some of the social sickness and alleviate some of the symptoms that afflicted the community as a whole. Unifying all against the one or the few prevented the disintegration of social ties that would lead to

---

[21] For what follows, see Jan Bremmer, "Scapegoat Rituals in Ancient Greece," in *The Oedipus Casebook: Reading Sophocles' Oedipus the King*, ed. Mark Rogin Anspach, Studies in Violence, Mimesis, and Culture (East Lansing: Michigan State University Press, 2020).
[22] See René Girard, *The Scapegoat*, Johns Hopkins Paperbacks ed. (Baltimore, MD: Johns Hopkins University Press, 1989).
[23] Rene Girard and Patrick Gregory, *Violence and the Sacred* (Baltimore, MD; London: Johns Hopkins University Press, 1977).

an each against each anarchy. Athenians had this treatment primed and ready, in their social medicine chest.

Scapegoating of this sort represents a specific conflation of medical and religious perspectives. As we saw above, we have an evolved biological revulsion for things that seem "impure" in health terms, even without any medical understanding of why they might be dangerous. This natural dynamic is intertwined with cultural and religious views of purity that bear more on maintaining social identities and boundaries. Both dimensions of purity, the biological and the social, can be mobilized or even fused to apply to groups or individuals already marginalized for other reasons.

If we return to the waves of plague in Christian Europe, we find a striking example. The advent of plague was often met with scapegoating violence against Jews. In the year 1349, hundreds of Jews were massacred by their neighbors in cities including Strasbourg, Erfurt, Zurich, and Basel.[24] Jews were accused of having spread the plague (poisoning wells or conveying infected goods). Or plague was seen as a punishment from God upon Christian countries for tolerating Jewish communities within them. Jews were accused with conveying biological contamination or with being themselves social contaminants. This is a virulently Christian version of the dynamic evident in the Athenian solution. In such contexts, social and political persecution takes on the character of a medical treatment.

Vaccines are among medicine's most dramatic achievements. They harness or train our own immune systems to resist infection from agents that produce horrific pandemics, such as smallpox. Introducing an attenuated or inactivated form of the virus, the vaccination prompts our immune system to produce the antibodies that will prevent us from developing the disease when exposed. One beneficial side effect of vaccines is that they have doubtless spared us not only from the direct ravages of these diseases but from the accompanying social violence and ostracism that would have accompanied those epidemics.

The sad truth is that scapegoating endures because it is also is effective. It does not cure illness. But it does reliably unite people who might otherwise be at odds with each other, by giving them a common enemy, a sense of agency against feared contamination, and a conviction of shared identity.

---

[24]Robert Steven Gottfried, *The Black Death: Natural and Human Disaster in Medieval Europe* (New York: Free Press; Collier Macmillan, 1983). 73ff. See also Samuel K. Cohn, "The Black Death and the Burning of Jews," *Past & Present* 196, no. 1 (2007): 3–36.

This security is reflected in the fact that no one who scapegoats views what they are doing as scapegoating. The action is understood as morally required and spiritually validated. It is not a close call. The more successful it is, the more it reinforces a sense of virtue and certainty.

One can be sure that these factors will be present in any serious epidemic. In the United States, we saw an initial reaction against Chinese or even Asian persons, a readiness to identify them at once as carriers of a virus that connected with another readiness to view them as a minority "contaminant" in society. We saw people, animated by fear of infection, willing to contemplate or endorse treatment of others they would have before automatically condemned as immoral: denial of medical treatment, forcible removal into camps. People on opposing sides of the "Covid wars," even when the question at issue was hardly clear in a medical sense, were ready to characterize each other in extreme terms, as threats to the health of the entire body of society.

From a Christian theological perspective, a primary epidemic-related task is precisely to monitor and articulate the religious resources relating to this dimension of the situation.[25] There is a central theological question, of which this is but one facet. Are the central tenets of Christian faith an incitement to scapegoating practice, or are they part of the immune resistance to it? As deployed at the personal, community, and cultural levels, do Christian beliefs and frameworks serve as part of a healthy immune system or do they become an autoimmune comorbidity?

As the medieval massacres of Jews described above make clear, Christians have demonstrated their capacity for the most virulent forms of scapegoating. And yet, as historian Tom Holland has pointed out, it is hard to account for our sensitivity to the issue itself apart from the cultural influence of the biblical tradition (from which we have taken the word).[26] "Scapegoat," as referring to an individual or minority *falsely and wrongly* condemned and punished by the unanimous agreement of our own community is a cultural and religious discovery, whose importance we must continually reappropriate. Our awareness that there is a scapegoat infection to resist has become part of our secular culture. This is good news, so that identifying it as an important concern in relation to epidemics need not be a specifically religious

---

[25]For more on scapegoating and theology, see S. Mark Heim, *Saved from Sacrifice: A Theology of the Cross* (Grand Rapids, MI: William B. Eerdmans Pub. Co., 2006).
[26]See Tom Holland, *Dominion: How the Christian Revolution Remade the World*, 1st US ed. (New York: Basic Books, 2019).

enterprise. But that sensibility is heir to a prior revolution, Holland says, one that has, "at its molten heart, the image of a god dead on a cross."[27]

At times—the civil rights movement in the United States would be an example—Christian sources have functioned precisely in this manner. Even when, initially, a majority of Christians resisted the movement for African American equality, that movement (led notably by ministers and predominantly based in Black churches) spoke from the deepest roots of that tradition. A religion based on God's identification with and vindication of the politically and religiously condemned victim is one that will always have resources to respond to this challenge. There is no greater contribution Christianity, in particular, can make to public health in plague times than to activate all its resources against the scapegoating autoimmune response.

Relevance of the Past

When we look back at epidemics, we realize that we have been here before. The Covid epidemic and the HIV epidemic (which we will consider in the next chapter) each have unique viral signatures, and our societies experienced these epidemics rather like random asteroid strikes. But the dynamics surrounding them, medical and social, have long been with us. William Faulkner once wrote, "The past is never dead. It isn't even past."[28]

Looking back at the impact of past epidemics, we can wonder about the future effects of those we have lived through, specifically on medicine and religion. Very quickly, we incorporated telehealth into our ambulatory settings and made our religious gatherings virtual. We became much nimbler than we ever thought we could be. How much will such changes lead to reimagined health care and religious practice going forward? We are beginning to come to grips with the spiritual and medical effects of prolonged isolation, with the impact on children of lost days of education and socialization, with the uneven economic deficits. We are facing the fallout from medical care and screenings that were deferred during the pandemic, and similar social and spiritual fallout from missed socialization and support.

---

[27]Ibid., 542.
[28]William Faulkner et al., *Requiem for a Nun* (New York: Random House, 1951), 73.

Pandemics bring out the best and worst in us. We can say this of religious traditions as much as of medical systems and political ones. During the Covid-19 pandemic, we read daily examples of heroism by healthcare workers, sacrifice by neighbors, and generosity of faith communities. But pandemics also touch on deep biological, social, and religious dispositions that can fuel scapegoating and division. This chapter lifts up themes around which medicine and religion can find common cause when, not if, we face such situations again.

References

Ayerst, David, and A.S.T. Fisher. *Records of Christianity*. 2 vols, vol. 1. Oxford: B. Blackwell, 1971.

Beck, Richard Allan. *Unclean: Meditations on Purity, Hospitality, and Morality*. Eugene, OR: Cascade Books, 2011.

Bremmer, Jan. "Scapegoat Rituals in Ancient Greece." In *The Oedipus Casebook: Reading Sophocles' Oedipus the King*, edited by Mark Rogin Anspach. Studies in Violence, Mimesis, and Culture, xiv, 459p. East Lansing: Michigan State University Press, 2020.

Cohn, Samuel K. "The Black Death and the Burning of Jews." [In English]. *Past & Present* 196, no. 1 (2007): 3–36.

Cunha, Burke A. *The Cause of the Plague of Athens: Plague, Typhoid, Typhus, Smallpox, or Measles?*, 29–43. Philadelphia: Elsevier Inc, 2004.

Faulkner, William, Meyer Wagman, William Faulkner, Herman Finkelstein Collection (Library of Congress), Ralph Ellison Collection (Library of Congress), Aramont Library Collection (Library of Congress), and Asprey & Co. *Requiem for a Nun*. New York: Random House, 1951.

Flick, Alexander Clarence. *The Decline of the Medieval Church*. Burt Franklin Bibliography & Reference Series,. New York: B. Franklin, 1967.

Getz, Faye Marie. "Black Death and the Silver Lining: Meaning, Continuity, and Revolutionary Change in Histories of Medieval Plague." *Journal of the History of Biology* 24, no. 2 (1991): 265–89.

Girard, René. *The Scapegoat*. Johns Hopkins paperbacks ed. Baltimore, MD: Johns Hopkins University Press, 1989.

Girard, Rene, and Patrick Gregory. *Violence and the Sacred*. Baltimore, MD; London: Johns Hopkins University Press, 1977.

Gottfried, Robert Steven. *The Black Death: Natural and Human Disaster in Medieval Europe*. New York London: Free Press; Collier Macmillan, 1983.

Heim, S. Mark. *Saved from Sacrifice: A Theology of the Cross.* Grand Rapids, MI: William B. Eerdmans Pub. Co., 2006.

Holland, Tom. *Dominion: How the Christian Revolution Remade the World.* First US edition. ed. New York: Basic Books, 2019.

Johnson, Paul. *A History of Christianity.* 1st American ed. New York: Atheneum, 1976.

Kadar, Nicholas, Roberto Romero, and Zoltán Papp. "Ignaz Semmelweis: The 'Savior of Mothers': On the 200th Anniversary of His Birth." [In English]. *American Journal of Obstetrics and Gynecology* 219, no. 6 (2018): 519–22.

Krieger, Nancy, Pamela D. Waterman, and Jarvis T. Chen. "Covid-19 and Overall Mortality Inequities in the Surge in Death Rates by Zip Code Characteristics: Massachusetts, January 1 to May 19, 2020." *American Journal of Public Health* 110, no. 12 (2020): 1850–2.

McNeill, William Hardy. *Plagues and Peoples.* 1st ed. Garden City, NY: Anchor Press, 1976.

Roberts, Carolyn. *To Heal and to Harm: Medicine, Knowledge, and Power in the Atlantic Slave Trade.* Cambridge, MA: Harvard University Press, 2017.

Savitt, Todd L. "Black Health on the Plantation: Owners, the Enslaved, and Physicians." *OAH Magazine of History* 19, no. 5 (2005): 14–16.

Shiode, Narushige, Shino Shiode, Elodie Rod-Thatcher, Sanjay Rana, and Peter Vinten-Johansen. "The Mortality Rates and the Space-Time Patterns of John Snow's Cholera Epidemic Map." [In English]. *International Journal of Health Geographics* 14, no. 1 (2015): 21–21.

Snowden, Frank M. *Epidemics and Society: From the Black Death to the Present.* The Open Yale Courses Series. New Haven, CT: Yale University Press, 2019.

Stark, Rodney. *The Rise of Christianity: How the Obscure, Marginal Jesus Movement Became the Dominant Religious Force in the Western World in a Few Centuries.* 1st HarperCollins pbk. ed. San Francisco, CA: HarperSanFrancisco, 1997.

Thucydides. *The Peloponnesian War.* Cambridge: Hackett, 1998.

Vrinten, C., A. Gallagher, J. Waller, and L.A.V. Marlow. "Cancer Stigma and Cancer Screening Attendance: A Population Based Survey in England." [In English]. *BMC Cancer* 19, no. 1 (2019): 566.

8

Stigma and Health
The HIV Epidemic

Chapter Outline

Rosa's Story	149
Worthy to be Well	152
We Are the Church, and the Church Has AIDS	154
Angels in America	157
Healed by Being Seen	160
Anxiety and Acceptance	162

Patients with HIV have been a major part of Ben's medical practice throughout his whole career, a time in which infection with HIV has gone from a near certain death sentence to a chronic condition that can be medically controlled. Nothing has affected him more than his interaction with those patients. This is his account of his journey with one of them, which we have left in the first person.

Rosa's Story

I met Rosa on the day she was diagnosed with HIV. She sat in a corner of my office. She clutched her sides and rocked slowly back and forth, chanting to herself, "I am going to die. I am going to die. I know I am going to die." She had just received her test results at the public health office and had been sent over to our practice.

Slowly, ever so gently, we listened—the nurse, the social worker, and I. Rosa shared that she had a young son. The father was in jail. Her employment was spotty. Life was hard before. Now a devastating diagnosis was just too much. "Who will take care of my son?" she asked.

Together, we stumbled through those first weeks, then months. By 1999, there were good HIV medications, and after a few weeks, the HIV virus was under control. Her immune system bounced back. And so did she. She no longer spoke of death. She gained weight. I became the doctor to her young son.

She started attending a church, a charismatic, storefront congregation. "When I'm at church," she said, "I just feel so good, so alive." She began to play the piano and teach the children. On another visit, she said, "I wanted to give up. I wanted to lose hope. But then God found me and saved me."

Years passed. She took her meds regularly. Our visits were mainly spent catching up about her adventures: her art projects, her church, her friends, her son. We would go over her labs, which had long ago demonstrated an undetectable viral load and a strong immune system. She brought in several of her drawings as gifts.

On one routine visit, she announced, "I stopped taking my pills."

"Why?" I asked, flummoxed, after so many years of good control.

"I believe that God has cured me of my HIV."

In my many years of practicing medicine and serving as a Christian pastor, I had never confronted a moment where the two sides of my life collided in quite that way. What could I say? I could not, in good conscience, affirm her belief that God had cured her of her HIV. With medications, the HIV viral load is controlled to undetectable levels. However, if a person stops her meds, the virus quickly rebounds, placing the person's health at great risk. But, I did not want to quash her optimism, her conviction. I did not want to alienate her from our practice, from modern medicine, from me.

"I just know that God has cured me," she affirmed with a joyful smile. I worried. Was she manic? Naive? In denial? The medication controlled her HIV, but it was her faith that restored her spirit, inspired her art, and gave her that vibrant smile. In a strange way, I wondered if she was being too prideful. God had singled *her* out? Who did she think she was?

"Do you ever pray?" I asked.

"Yes, all the time," she said."

Do you ever pray with other people?" I asked.

"Yes, at church, all the time," she said.

"Would you mind if we prayed together right now?" I asked.

"Of course! I would love that doc," she said.

And so we did, a simple, brief prayer that God would keep her healthy, keep her safe. . . and keep her coming back. She agreed to recurrent visits, every three months, to check her viral load and her immune system. I could not, in good conscience, prescribe medications that she would never take. If she took the medications inconsistently, the virus could become resistant, making future regimens more difficult.

True to her word, she returned regularly. We checked labs. We talked about her kid, her church, her friends, her art. Amazingly, her viral load remained undetectable for several years—which I really cannot explain. Once, I even clicked the box to recheck her HIV antibody test. Maybe she *was* cured? At each visit, we discussed that, at some point, the HIV virus would return, and her immune system would weaken. She would nod in agreement, as if to appease me. We would close our visits in prayer.

Bit by bit, the HIV virus crept back. 50 copies. . . 187 copies. . . 1,500 copies. I became more earnest in our conversations. Her T-cells began to drift downwards, an indication that her immune system was weakening. 600. . . 457. . . 378. By then, we had covered a lot of ground together: medical, personal, spiritual.

In the end, Rosa began taking her medications again with a renewed commitment. She had reframed her illness. HIV was a chronic disease, not a source of shame. She reframed her faith. These medications were a gift from God, which would empower her life to serve, to grow, to live. These medications would keep her alive if she took them regularly. In its own way, her journey modeled what Anselm of Canterbury proposed, "Faith seeking understanding." In this case, her faith had been seeking the way to understand her illness and respond to it. Her faith and her approach to medicine were no longer opposed. Her viral load quickly became undetectable. Her immune system rebounded. She continues to be healthy and to serve in her church.

Ben's experience with Rosa illustrated what he has come to call his first law of medicine: "The Medicine Is Easy. Everything Else Is Hard." It is easy to write a prescription for a once a day medication with minimal side effects that is most assuredly able to control this deadly disease. The art of medicine, the healing, is for the patient to discover for themselves that the medication can save their lives. Sometimes this takes reframing the narrative of illness and health. It takes patience, trust, and love.

HIV is particularly challenging for patients because so often the infection is accompanied by shame or guilt. HIV is often contracted through unprotected intercourse or sharing needles when injecting drugs. In the early days, blood transfusions were another mode of transmission, which was quickly rectified. The control of the illness is easy: take the medication. However, the turmoil of the spirit is more challenging.

Worthy to be Well

In Ben's HIV practice, he has noticed that patients have two different approaches to medications. For many, the medications are a pathway to health. Most patients take the medications most of the time. These days, there are new formulations where three drugs are contained in one pill. The three drugs have minimal side effects. However, some identify the medications with the stigma of their disease. The medications remind them of who they slept with or their drug use. What is the cure for shame? Guilt? The nagging feeling that maybe you deserved your lot in life?

Rosa's story presented the question of how to convince someone to take a medicine she wholeheartedly believes she do not need to take. But it is often a case of trying to convince someone to take a medicine when they don't think they deserve to be healed. Ben worries that some patients punish themselves because they feel that they are not worthy of care. It is easy to order a blood test or a CT scan. But it is hard to instill hope when a patient has lost it. It is especially hard during a 20-minute visit when there are other patients waiting in the next exam rooms.

Shame is a complicated spiritual condition. Shame can derive from one's own intrinsic belief systems. Did I deserve this? More often, shame is imposed by the complex structures of society. Moral judgment upon those with HIV has been cruel. Many people with HIV know this sentiment of other-ness and alienation from those they love and society at large. To unwind the harm takes strong spiritual care. The only cure for shame is love. As HIV can be controlled with medications that suppress the virus, so too can shame be kept at bay with love. If we stop taking the medications, the virus returns. The same can be true of spiritual supports that keep shame, guilt and despair in check.

The collisions that occurred in Ben's office had been happening on a larger, much less gentle scale across our country and the world. AIDS (as it was then called) was at first most effectively spread by means of male-to-male sexual relations and intravenous drug use, activities already stigmatized in society. This gave ample fodder for those not immediately associated with such activities to condemn the victims for their own affliction. Christianity figured in that cultural moment primarily as the source of religious ammunition to support that hateful indifference. Many churches and Christian leaders said directly or indirectly that the ravages of HIV were a divine punishment for prior immoral behaviors. Roman Catholics, who opposed artificial means of birth control, maintained their opposition to condoms, although they offered a barrier to transmission of HIV to those not yet infected.

In this environment, HIV-positive people often felt the need to keep their status secret for fear of discrimination. They might be ostracized or forced out of their churches, even their families. At a time when they faced the most devastating illness and all the stress that went with it, they were deprived of their existing social and spiritual resources. Those with strong personal faith, which would be a support in such a time, might feel that they were losing that along with their religious community.

With contagious disease, moral and spiritual hazards are close at every hand. When everyone is equally at risk, that undifferentiated fear gives rise to the scapegoating dynamic we discussed in the previous chapter. We saw that great plagues of history made little distinction, killing those in all stations and stages of life. Where disease makes no medical distinction, humans labor to create or find a social or moral one, identifying some as guilty parties and uniting against them. That instinct seeks to find one or a few as responsible for the disease, against whom a reassuring unanimity can be constituted.

But when the contagious disease has sharply differentiated risk and affects a definable minority, we readily make that minority culpable for their own illness. We conflate some other moral or social hierarchy with the actual profile of the epidemic. HIV disproportionately affected persons who already were socially marginalized, skewing the public health response through pre-existing prejudices. Covid, on the other hand, most severely affected the oldest among us, and on a scale that made it hard to treat them as an isolated group.

Both HIV and Covid presented public health with decisions that were not purely medical. Officials had to thread a needle in responding not just to the clinical issues of infection and treatment but also to the social and spiritual forms of contagion. Many in the gay community criticized the public messaging around HIV for not directly addressing the communities most at risk and stressing the particular responses that might best protect them (for instance, safer sex or injection practices). But some in public health felt medical and research resources could not be mobilized unless the threat was perceived to extend to the general population. When everyone feels at risk, the fear levels can lead to mistaken policy. But when most people feel secure, it is all too easy to regard the suffering of others as their problem alone. It is difficult to "treat" an epidemic without considering the contagion not only of viruses but of fear and social and religious imagery.

We Are the Church, and the Church Has AIDS

In the early years of the HIV epidemic, Mark had an opportunity to be closely connected with the Universal Fellowship of Metropolitan Community Churches—a newly formed Christian community in the United States unequivocally inclusive of lesbian and gay persons.[1] At the time, HIV was still peripheral in general public awareness, but negative characterizations and religious condemnation were already clearly in play. In that setting, the UFMCC churches presented a startlingly different pattern. The communion was founded by people of strong faith—often leaders in their former churches—who had been excluded from those communities because of their sexual orientation. It had become a refuge for such exiles. It was also a creative spiritual renewal movement, fueled by the wide variety of prior traditions its members brought with them, and which otherwise would never have mixed so vibrantly.

Begun in 1968, all the UFMCC then had time to do, one of its founders said, "was to celebrate and grow."[2] But in a few years the AIDS crisis thrust these young churches into a maelstrom of personal and communal suffering.

---

[1] He was a member of the Faith and Order Commission of the National Council of Churches. The UFMCCC had applied for membership in the National Council, and its application had been referred to the commission for study. As a result, he spent several years in close dialogue with pastors and members from these churches, as they were grappling with the early stages of the epidemic.

[2] Kittredge Cherry and James Mitulski, "We Are the Church Alive, the Church with AIDS. (Metropolitan Community Church of San Francisco)," 105, no. 3 (1988): 86, https://go.exlibris.link /jL2B4WLc.

The UFMCC was especially strong in the San Francisco area, ground zero for the HIV epidemic. Its members and congregations were immersed in care for those who were sick and dying. In the early years of the epidemic, when victims were often held at arm's length even by medical institutions, the community of the afflicted became a spiritual movement in its own right. Gay people and their loved ones bonded together to provide each other what doctors, churches, and even families so often failed to offer: loving support up to and through death, rituals of lament and remembrance, guerilla forms of medical research and treatment, political agitation. By virtue of its openness as an affirming religious space, the UFMCC became a center of spiritual support for victims of the disease.

One UFMCC congregation dealing with HIV death after death among its members still found itself growing by a third each year. Its pastors said it had been thrust into a form of "eschatological living" where grief contended with new and intense forms of spiritual growth and community. Each month, it celebrated funerals for people who had never entered its sanctuary, but whose family and friends had come because they would not be welcomed in their own home churches.

Even while the theological response of many Christian groups (because of negative attitudes toward same-sex relations) played a destructive role in the crisis, there were also points of light. Some Roman Catholic hospices and hospitals were among those few traditional caregivers on the medical front lines, animated by mercy and compassion above all. The UFMCC became a natural networking point for Christians in other denominations to connect with each other.[3]

It is hard to imagine a population for whom religion would seem less likely to enhance health than the gay communities suffering so profoundly from HIV. Many of them were estranged from their religious backgrounds or had been actively driven from those communities. Yet a review of studies from 1980 to 2016 evaluating the association between religion, spirituality, and clinical outcomes for HIV-infected persons (such as T-cell counts, viral load, mortality) showed a surprisingly positive relation.[4] Large proportions (ranging from 65 percent to 85 percent, using different measures) of HIV patients indicated that religion and spirituality were important in their lives

---

[3] See Letty M. Russell, *The Church with Aids: Renewal in the Midst of Crisis*, 1st ed. (Louisville, KY: Westminster/John Knox Press, 1990).
[4] B.R. Doolittle, A.C. Justice, and D.A. Fiellin, "Religion, Spirituality, and HIV Clinical Outcomes: A Systematic Review of the Literature," *AIDS and Behavior* 22, no. 6 (2018): 1792–801.

and in their response to their illness. Two-thirds of the studies indicated religion and spiritual involvement correlated with better health outcomes in the progression of the disease.

A few of the studies provided some indication of the specific forms of religious involvement that were associated with more negative outcomes. One showed men who have sex with men and attend church regularly presented with lower T-cell counts (i.e., more advanced disease) at their first medical intake, suggesting that they resisted recognizing their condition. In such cases, religious involvement appeared to be associated with denial of symptoms, perhaps out of fear of stigma. Another study indicated those who viewed God as predominantly punishing and judgmental rather than benevolent and forgiving experienced more rapid disease progression.[5] Despite the special challenges faced by HIV positive people, spiritual engagement still remained a key factor in their medical conditions.

One event in particular stood out for Mark, an ecumenical Lenten worship service he attended in San Francisco in the spring of 1989, whose theme was "We Have AIDS." The sermon was preached by Rev. Ron Russell-Coons, who was himself dying of the virus.[6] He began by unflinchingly describing himself in the language of Paul's letter to the Corinthians: "Therefore, we do not lose heart. Though outwardly we are wasting away, yet inwardly we are being renewed day by day."[7] He recognized the message coming from many Christian pulpits, to the effect that those with HIV deserved what they received, that they were "throw away people." But for God, he affirmed, there were no throw away people. We belong to the church, he said. We have AIDS. "We are the church, and the church has AIDS."

When AIDS was still often a closeted condition, even within an already stigmatized gay community that faced the reality every day, this was a startling confession. It was both an admission and a witness. It acknowledged the illness without hesitation. And it claimed the apostle Paul's confession that all the members of the church are one body, the body of Christ. What one part of the body has, all have. The body of Christ had AIDS. Some of us had the disease in body. Some of us had it in the form of grief and loss. Some of us had it in a particularly virulent form of hard-heartedness and fear toward others. This meant it was not the concern of some of us, but of all.

---

[5] Gail Ironson et al., "View of God as Benevolent and Forgiving or Punishing and Judgmental Predicts HIV Disease Progression," *Journal of Behavioral Medicine* 34, no. 6 (2011): 414–25.
[6] Ron Russell-Coons, "We Have Aids."
[7] 2 Corinthians 4:16.

The theology behind that proclamation was impeccable. Unfortunately, it was not typical of Christian churches or other communities. The challenge for religious traditions and communities in plague times is to emphasize the expression of their unique resources for building inclusive social environments, the dimensions of faith that impel us into care for the whole and for neighbors in the most concrete sense. The UFMCC demonstrated how this could be done

Angels in America

Religion and medicine collided very publicly with the play *Angels in America*, one of the most celebrated plays in Broadway history, winning the 1993 Tony for Best Play, as well as a raft of other awards. *Angels* wrestles with the HIV epidemic of the mid-1980s through the eyes of four main characters in two couples: a conservative gay lawyer with his delusional wife (both Mormons) and a gay man dying of AIDS with his faithless male lover. The play was not without controversy, related partly to its frank gay sexuality and direct treatment of religious hostility to homosexuality. It is suffused with Mormon and Jewish religious imagery. Alongside the four human protagonists, a cast of supernatural beings, angels, weaves in and out of the story, as though the author is seeking some wider religious landscape into which the plot of HIV can be mapped. Indeed, the drama's primary theme is to superimpose a hallucinatory millennial apocalypse over 1980s New York City, with HIV as the final plague.

In one of the last scenes in the play, God is indicted for abandoning humanity to the epidemic and all other suffering: ". . . if he did come back, you should *sue* the bastard. That's my only contribution to all this theology. Sue the bastard for walking out."[8] And yet the very final scene evokes a different kind of end-of-the-world vision, one in which a healing fountain will be opened in which everyone can be immersed and made whole. "We will all bathe ourselves clean."[9]

One narrative arc in the play links the well-connected, unscrupulous lawyer Roy Cohn and his Black, gay nurse, Belize. Cohn is a closeted gay

---

[8]Tony Kushner, *Angels in America: A Gay Fantasia on National Themes*, 1st ed., 2 vols., vol. 2 (New York: Theatre Communications Group, 1993), 133.
[9]Ibid., 145–8.

man, hospitalized and dying from HIV. Belize cares for him on the night shift.

There is a scene where Roy Cohn asks, "Can I ask you something sir? What's it like, after?" [10]

> "After?" says Belize
> "This misery ends...." responds Cohn.
> "Hell or heaven?"
> "heh...." says Cohn. The playwright is deliberately vague. Does Cohn mean "heaven" or "hell?"
> "Like San Francisco"
> "A city, good," says Cohn, "I was worried it would be a garden. I hate that shit."
> "A big city, overgrown with weeds but flowering weeds," continues Belize. On every corner a wrecking crew and something new and crooked going up kitty corner to that. Windows missing in every edifice like broken teeth, gritty wind and a gray, high sky full of ravens . . . piles of trash but lapidary like rubies and obsidian and diamond colored cowspit streamers in the wind and voting booths and everyone in Balenciaga gowns with red corsages, big dance palaces full of music, lights and racial impurity and gender confusion and all the deities are Creole, mulatto, brown as the mouths of rivers . . . race . . . taste . . . and history, finally overcome. And you ain't there.
> "And heaven?" Roy asks.
> "That was heaven...."

Belize inverts the contemporary power structure. Cohn is wealthy and powerful, but also dying and alone. Belize is the night shift, Black nurse, the bottom of the health care power structure. Yet, throughout, Belize conveys wisdom, faithfulness, and genuine care, despite the abusive tirades Cohn directs at him.

In the scene, the play powerfully demonstrates how HIV brings together those who would otherwise have little to do with each other and little care for each other. The conversation is set within the fraught dynamics of the medical system. Belize warns Cohn to avoid the radiation his doctor is recommending, as it will make his condition worse. When he asks why he should believe her rather than his expensive doctor, he replies "He's not queer. I am."[11] Cohn has used influence to get into a trial study of the new AIDS drug AZT, and Belize coaches him on how to be sure he gets the drug

---

[10] For what follows, ibid., 77–8.
[11] Ibid., 29.

and not a placebo. All of this is doubtless knowledge she has gained through the underground activism of patient support groups. In these respects, her care for him as a fellow sufferer outweighs her distaste for his politics and morals. Just as at the individual level faith and medicine can reinforce each other or conflict, so at the community level, religious beliefs and practices can foster common concern for healing or can undermine it by isolating people from each other's suffering.

Kushner's play overflows with references from the Bible and Jewish tradition. The scene between Cohn and Belize is echoed in the Hebrew Bible in 2 Kgs 5:1-19. That passage tells the story of General Naaman, the most powerful military leader of the Arameans and an enslaved girl whom he captured in a raid against Israel. General Namaan has it all: power, wealth, and prestige. And yet, he hides a secret: he has leprosy. In the ancient world, leprosy was more than a life-threatening disease. It was also a mark of sin and shame. The ultimate power broker, the ultimate insider, was in fact the ultimate outsider. General Namaan is the Roy Cohn of the Hebrew Bible.

Enter an unnamed, enslaved girl who belongs to an enemy people. Her name has been lost to history. She is dispossessed, at the mercy of her captor, for whom we would expect her to have only hatred. Nevertheless, she has pity on the general. To Namaan's wife, she says, "If only my lord were before the prophet who is in Samaria! Then he would take away his leprosy from him."[12]

Naaman uses money to persuade the King of Israel to allow him to present his case to the prophet Elisha. But when he goes to the prophet, Elisha does not even deign to greet the General at his door, but instead commands him to wash seven times in the river Jordan. The General is non-plussed at this treatment and his pride offended. Are not there rivers in Damascus and yet he is required to bathe in a foreign river? Reluctantly, the General washes in the river Jordan and is healed.

This ancient story, which has a clipped, spare tone, is about grace and power. General Namaan's earthly power was an illusion, just as Roy Cohn's was. The real healing comes from grace, unmerited love, as modeled by Belize and the enslaved girl. Was there healing on the night shift between Cohn and Belize? Cohn still dies a painful death from his disease. But in their exchange, in Belize's tough-love tenderness, we see a glimmer of the solidarity that grows up in such suffering.

---

[12] 2 Kings 5:3.

Kushner's play is a testimony to the links between medical and religious discourse. Kushner grapples with the enormity of the suffering caused by the HIV epidemic, the indifference of much of society, and with the fear that the entire story of the struggle and despair, but also the beauty and nobility that HIV engendered in the gay community would vanish culturally without a trace. In his passionate commitment to affirm the meaning of that story and the dignity of the wounded people in it, he reaches naturally to weave it into the spiritual sources in whose terms we have framed our most profound experiences of suffering and of redemption.

Healed by Being Seen

Angels in America looks back at a time when a medical cure or treatment for HIV was only a hope, and the only forms of healing possible required solidarity, love, and spiritual support. All of those things often had to be sought apart from or even against the grain of existing medical and religious institutions. Medical education increasingly recognizes the significance of these factors.

One of the most prestigious events at the Yale Medical School is the Yale Department of Medicine Grand Rounds. Usually, Grand Rounds is a formal lecture, where a faculty member presents leading research. It is a time of formality and highly polished presentations. Yet, once a year it is devoted to a "story slam," where the subject is not clinical research but the lived experience of healing. Members from across the Yale community submit dozens of stories and only a handful are chosen to be read at Grand Rounds, before an audience of several hundred people. It is always the most highly attended Grand Rounds of the year, and quite an honor to be selected to be one of the presenters.

Karina Danvers was one so chosen, and we have taken every opportunity to have her share her story with our students. For many years, she was the director of a large education program for HIV providers. She came to be known by physicians and nurses as a colleague, an expert on the disease, and an activist in public outreach and in the education of health care workers. But she did not come to the Grand Rounds to talk about her professional activities. She came to report what it means to be a patient. For Karina is HIV positive.

When she was first diagnosed in the 1990s, she remembers going into the hospital for a routine procedure, which required an intravenous line to be placed. "You know I'm HIV positive," she said to the nurse. "I know," the nurse nervously replied. In the moment when the IV was put in place, a small drop of blood fell from Karina's arm on to the floor. "You would have thought there was an outbreak of the plague," she says. Environmental control was called. Maintenance staff showed up with mops and buckets. Gallons of bleach were used to disinfect the area. Karina watched this frantic activity, feeling more and more what it meant to be regarded as a threat, as the source of a dangerous disease, as someone feared.

She is candid and vulnerable in recounting what it was like to come to terms with her illness, or to be unable to. "I remember when the only thing I wanted was to kill myself, but at the same time to live," she said. "I remember coming out of the HIV closet and speaking at schools, clinics, and hospitals," she continued. "Kids and adults were stunned that AIDS looked like me—a married, working, heterosexual, non-IV-drug-using woman."[13] She struggled against the impulse to separate herself from other HIV patients, as an "innocent one," who had not acquired the virus in the manner people assumed. She does not present her story as one with a simple or happy ending. "In a way, I have come to peace with my HIV, but it has been incredibly hard."

Danvers was raised as an active Catholic. Faith is important to her. She has appreciated support from priests and the life of the church. But here too it has often been hard for others in her religious community to appreciate her spiritual struggle. When she looked back over her experience with HIV, she said one of her deepest sadnesses was that none of the health care workers that cared for her had ever said, "I am sorry." I am sorry that this has happened. I am sorry that you have to go through this. One of our students asked her if that was something she would like to hear from God. In tears, she agreed. "I have wanted to hear 'I'm sorry', from God. 'I'm sorry that you are suffering.'"

The evolution of treatment for HIV meant that, medically, Karina Danvers' condition became more stable and more hopeful. But the meaning of her disease and her experience of it included much that still required

---

[13]For the quotations from Danvers in this paragraph, see Riley Davis, "Grand Rounds: Telling Stories Is Fundamental to Being a Physician," *Yale School of Medicine*, https://medicine.yale.edu/news-article/grand-rounds-telling-stories-is-fundamental-to-being-a-physician/.

reconciliation and resolution. It was that kind of healing, healing from isolation, rejection, and self-doubt that she set out to help others attain as she sought it herself.

Anxiety and Acceptance

We have seen that one of the dramatic comorbidities for HIV, one of the things that increased the suffering of the disease and undercut well-being for its victims, was alienation. Simply by virtue of becoming sick, and so in even greater need of support and meaning, HIV patients were often rejected by or estranged from the very networks of family, social supports, and religious community that normally enhance health. In this case, that estrangement was the circumstantial response to a specific disease. But philosophers and theologians often diagnosis and address this issue in a more universal sense: occasions of suffering uncover something we have otherwise been able to ignore or deny.

Jean Paul Sartre and Simone de Beauvoir articulated this in their versions of existentialism. One of their core principles was that existence itself is a state of anxiety. "It is certain that we cannot escape anguish," says Sartre, "for we are anguish."[14] This perspective was informed by the wanton destruction and the callous, devaluing of life during the Second World War. "Nothingness lies coiled at the heart of being like a worm," Sartre said, capturing the despairing spirit of the post-war generation. [15]

Much of this anxiety derived from what Sartre called *le regard*, the gaze. When another looks at you, you sense this observation and respond by feeling anxious, anxious about how one will be judged, anxious for the other's good opinion. "The Other's look," Sartre writes, "fashions my body in its nakedness, causes it to be born, sculptures it, produces it as it *is* . . . The Other holds a secret—the secret of *what I am*"[16] In the gaze, the Other is objectified, vulnerable, stripped away from social convention. In this helpless exposure, there is only apprehension and fear. From this perspective, one

---

[14] Jean-Paul Sartre, *Existentialism Is a Humanism* (New Haven, CT: Yale University Press, 2007), 29.
[15] Jean-Paul Sartre, *Being and Nothingness: An Essay on Phenomenological Ontology* (Paris: Gallimard, 1943), 21.
[16] Jean-Paul Sartre, *Being and Nothingness: An Essay on Phenomenological Ontology* (New York: Washington Square Press, 1968). 475.

deep anguish for those ill with HIV (or something else) is the regard with which they feel others regarding them, regarding them as a hostile or rejected "them."

Martin Buber, the celebrated Jewish existential philosopher, countered this sentiment in his work, *I and Thou*. Buber describes two relationships, *I-it* and *I-thou*.[17] In the *I-it* relationship, the subject regards the Other as an object. Such a gaze has all the alienating potential for the recipient that Sartre suggests. But in Buber's I-thou relationship, there is no impermeable boundary between the self and the Other. Each participates in the other, as subject and not only as an object. The I-thou relationship is the one between the Self and God and so, potentially between all persons.

Buber argues that we long to have a presence within the other. "Secretly and bashfully" we watch for "a YES which ... can come only from one human person to another."[18] What if *le regard* were not a gaze of judgement that resulted in anxiety? What if *le regard* were a gaze of recognition and acceptance?

Sickness intensifies this fundamental human tension between anxiety and acceptance: in medical contexts, we have simply tuned it to a particular frequency. It is a frequency that can be an avenue of healing (as we discussed in Chapter 4), or it can make every medical challenge into a new occasion of alienation and distress. For a patient, an I-it relation is to be treated only as a body or a disease. An I-thou relation is to be recognized as a person.

In the medical context, love does not demand intimacy or deep emotional commitment between caregivers and patients. In line with Buber's thought, we can think of love simply as a responsibility, the responsibility of any I for a thou, if the relation is to maintain its mutuality. In Chapter 2, in discussing both ministry and medicine as callings, we recalled Levinas' description of the sense of obligation that is communicated in the face of another person. The imperative we had in view there was the imperative to help, with special medical or religious training held not as a private possession, but as gifts in trust for others. Buber's vision supplements this with something that is not vocational, but existential. It belongs to the healing relationship simply as it preserves its quality as a human relation.

---

[17]Martin Buber, *I and Thou*, 2nd ed. (New York: Scribner, 1958).
[18]Martin Buber, *The Martin Buber Reader: Essential Writings*, ed. Asher D. Biemann (New York: Palgrave Macmillan, 2002), 212.

This is where the language of theology helps ground a vision of healing and reconciliation. Buber's I-thou is clearly based on a divine pattern. The human realization of that relation may be episodic. But God's relation with us constantly embodies it. A core principle of Christianity is the concept of *Imago Dei*, the conviction that we are made in the image of God. The theologian Irenaeus amplified this to say that we are made in the "image and likeness" of God.[19] By "image," he meant an indelible and irreversible dignity that belonged to us as gift, even when we entirely fail to live up to it. By "likeness," he meant the possibility of divine similarity that we could grow into, as for instance in realizing the I-thou relation with God and others more fully.

Medical practice has come to adopt standards for medical care that apply more to the relation with patients than their biological treatment—ideals like patient autonomy and informed consent. These are admirable principles, born of a recognition that therapeutic treatment should not override the dignity of the person concerned. But they ultimately must rest on a deeper foundation than mere prescription, within those who honor them. For Christians, the idea of the image of God expresses this conviction in a universal way, even as the invitation to see Christ presented to us in each encounter with our neighbor expresses it in a very religiously particular way.

If there is any moral to our review of the HIV epidemic, it is the importance of the gaze with which we attend to those who are ill (including the gaze we cast on ourselves when we are ill). That regard, something that we are exquisitely tuned to register and appropriate, works powerfully to heal or harm. One dimension of spirituality is simply the disciplines and practices for nurturing what is life-giving in this ecology of mutual regard. These practices shape the fundamental way in which we sense ourselves to be seen, at our deepest and most vulnerable core. The divine regard toward us, which Christians often call grace, comes from one who has an unobstructed view of that core, and who communicates an unequivocal will for our good. Faith, the response to that regard, has one bedrock feature that is always medically significant, whether our disease is cured or not: the conviction that we are all worthy to be healed.

---

[19] See J. Patout Burns et al., *Theological Anthropology*, Revised and Expanded ed., Ad Fontes: Early Christian Sources (Minneapolis, MN: Fortress Press, 2023), 23–8.

References

Buber, Martin. *I and Thou*. 2nd ed. New York: Scribner, 1958.
Buber, Martin. *The Martin Buber Reader: Essential Writings*. Edited by Asher D. Biemann. New York: Palgrave Macmillan, 2002.
Burns, J. Patout, Joseph Wilson Trigg, Robin Darling Young, and Jeffrey Thomas Wickes. *Theological Anthropology*. [Translated from the original languages into English.] Ad Fontes: Early Christian Sources. Revised and expanded ed. Minneapolis, MN: Fortress Press, 2023.
Cherry, Kittredge, and James Mitulski. "We Are the Church Alive, the Church with Aids. (Metropolitan Community Church of San Francisco)." 105, no. 3 (1988): 85. https://go.exlibris.link/jL2B4WLc.
Davis, Riley. "Grand Rounds: Telling Stories Is Fundamental to Being a Physician." *Yale School of Medicine*. https://medicine.yale.edu/news-article/grand-rounds-telling-stories-is-fundamental-to-being-a-physician/.
Doolittle, B.R., A.C. Justice, and D.A. Fiellin. "Religion, Spirituality, and HIV Clinical Outcomes: A Systematic Review of the Literature." [In English]. *AIDS and Behavior* 22, no. 6 (2018): 1792–801.
Ironson, Gail, Rick Stuetzle, Dale Ironson, Elizabeth Balbin, Heidemarie Kremer, Annie George, Neil Schneiderman, and Mary Ann Fletcher. "View of God as Benevolent and Forgiving or Punishing and Judgmental Predicts HIV Disease Progression." [In English]. *Journal of Behavioral Medicine* 34, no. 6 (2011): 414–25.
Kushner, Tony. *Angels in America : A Gay Fantasia on National Themes*. 1st ed. 2 vols. New York: Theatre Communications Group, 1993.
Russell, Letty M. *The Church with Aids: Renewal in the Midst of Crisis*. 1st ed. Louisville, KY: Westminster/John Knox Press, 1990.
Russell-Coons, Ron. "We Have Aids." In *The Church with AIDS: Renewal in the Midst of Crisis*, edited by Letty M. Russell, 35–45. Louisville, KY: Westminster/John Knox Press, 1990.
Sartre, Jean-Paul. *Being and Nothingness; An Essay on Phenomenological Ontology*. New York: Washington Square Press, 1968.

9

Addiction Therapy of Hope and Forgiveness

Chapter Outline

A Treatment That Looks Like a Church	170
Medical Models	174
Forgiveness as a Health Issue	178

In this chapter and the next, we consider two conditions of special interest because of their significance when it is doctors and ministers who are themselves the patients. Care givers are of course liable to any medical condition. But certain illnesses are of particular concern in regard to certain professions. Pilots, physicians, clergy, health care workers all have responsibilities such that their impairment can have serious consequences for those they care for. Addiction and burnout stand out in this connection, as disabilities that can undercut the very therapeutic skills that may be used to cure or ameliorate them. These afflictions are of special concern in both the care givers we are focused on, and in both afflictions the strands of religion and medicine are wound together very closely.

Addiction has always evoked "crossover" reflections, drawing attention from philosophy, psychology, and theology as well as medicine. In part, this is because addiction is complex. It is a disorder of goods. What drives addiction is an attraction to subjective states of being which are goods in themselves: bliss, relaxation, heightened sensation, relief from pain. These are neither evil nor destructive except in their relative power to overwhelm responsibility, relation, and deeper life goals. That power can crowd out any complementary good, laying waste to lives. The result is a permanent-feeling internal battle, between the me who chooses the substance above all else, and the me who, even almost at the same moment, longs for an alternate life. There could hardly be a more concrete expression of Paul's complaint in the book of Romans, "I do not understand what I do. For what I want to do I do not do, but what I hate I do . . . For I have the desire to do what is good, but I cannot carry it out. For I do not do the good I want to do, but the evil I do not want to do—this I keep on doing."[1] Christian groups have long debated in theological theory the relative mix of external grace and internal effort required for liberation from conditions like this, addiction in this respect being but a tangible face of a reality shared by all.

A psychiatrist and neurologist recently told a meeting of Mark's divinity school faculty that in his view it was widely recognized among his colleagues that a medically reductive approach to psychiatry had failed. It had failed across the board, although in two areas he believed the field had made major strides toward reversing this error and recognizing the therapeutic role of spirituality and religion: palliative care (primarily end of life) and addiction studies. It is not surprising to hear this assessment from a psychiatrist, for in both mental illness and addiction it is our meaning and decision-making faculties themselves that are affected, impaired. And it those same faculties that must be deployed by both the care giver and the patient as resources for healing.

In such a paradoxical condition, where health requires a transformation in our basic capacities, it is not easy to sharply distinguish treatment from a kind of conversion. The very instrumental means by which a medical treatment can be carried out—the intentions and decisions that lead to patients taking the medicine as prescribed, keeping appointments, maintaining a diet or therapy—are what is out of order. The very forms of ideation, social connection, and ritual regulation, through which religious faith plays a role in shaping and supporting persons, themselves become disrupted or distorted. This catch-22 becomes a common ground between religion and medicine, where both search for a source of transformation that

---

[1] Romans 7:15–19.

must arise from within the very thoughts and perceptions that are themselves disordered.

One Yale psychiatrist has devoted his research to people who literally hear voices.[2] According to his estimates something on the order of 15 percent of the population hear voices either regularly or episodically. Only a small portion of that group (something like a tenth of them) receive a specific mental health diagnosis indicating need for treatment or serious dysfunction. Rather than focusing on the causation and treatment of that smaller, medically prominent group, the psychiatrist was interested in understanding the rest. What made those people able to live more effectively and even happily with this phenomenon? His conclusion was that it had in great measure to do with the spiritual and religious context in which they understood the voices and related to them. His population of interest was people who, usually through no intention or effort of their own, heard an audible (as opposed to imagined) voice speaking to them. Tanya Luhrman's fascinating book *When God Talks Back*, dealt with a population in rather the reverse context: evangelical Christians who were seeking to cultivate an awareness of God speaking to them, despite the fact that their normal experience was totally devoid of such phenomena.[3] These mirror images illumine a landscape in which mental and spiritual health share one complex ecosystem of interpretive meaning.

Lying at the intersection of morality, philosophy, religion, psychology, and medicine, addiction has generated many interpretive and therapeutic models. Until the last century, addiction was primarily viewed not as a medical problem but as a psychological or a moral failing. That is, the medical response to addiction tended to appeal to categories of character or will. The treatments that corresponded to such diagnoses—extended psychological analysis, moral instruction, religious prayers for deliverance—proved notoriously ineffective on the whole.

---

[2] Albert R. Powers, Claire Bien, and Philip R. Corlett, "Aligning Computational Psychiatry with the Hearing Voices Movement: Hearing Their Voices," *JAMA Psychiatry (Chicago, Ill.)* 75, no. 6 (2018): 640–1; See also Tanya M. Luhrmann et al., "Learning to Discern the Voices of Gods, Spirits, Tulpas, and the Dead," *Schizophrenia Bulletin* 49, no. Supplement_1 (2023): S3–S12.
[3] T.M. Luhrmann, *When God Talks Back: Understanding the American Evangelical Relationship with God*, 1st ed. (New York: Alfred A. Knopf, 2012).

A Treatment That Looks Like a Church

One of the great contributions of the spiritual to the medical realms in the last century remade the treatment of addiction. This was Alcoholics Anonymous (AA), started in the 1930s by Bill Wilson and Bob Smith. AA meetings originated as refuges, at a time when those seeking assistance from either medical or religious figures were likely to encounter little more than exhortation and condemnation. AA gave rise to several offshoots dealing with issues from narcotics to gambling. A recent study indicated that 73 percent of addiction treatment programs in the United States "include a spirituality-based element, as embodied in the programs and fellowships initially popularized by Alcoholics Anonymous."[4] These "12 step" programs have operated out of church basements, community centers, and medical clinic conference rooms, serving millions in numberless locations.

The program revolves around the twelve steps, which are a cross between a creed, a diagnosis, a treatment regimen, and a life philosophy.[5] They are designed to guide a person struggling with addiction through a process of reconciliation with others, with oneself, and with a higher power. The steps were explicitly formulated in a Christian context, and make liberal reference

---

[4] Brian J. Grim and Melissa E. Grim, "Belief, Behavior, and Belonging: How Faith Is Indispensable in Preventing and Recovering from Substance Abuse," *Journal of Religion and Health* 58 (2019): 1713.
[5] The twelve steps are as follows:

1. We admitted we were powerless over alcohol—that our lives had become unmanageable.
2. Came to believe that a power greater than ourselves could restore us to sanity.
3. Made a decision to turn our will and our lives over to the care of God as we understood Him.
4. Made a searching and fearless moral inventory of ourselves.
5. Admitted to God, to ourselves, and to another human being the exact nature of our wrongs.
6. Were entirely ready to have God remove all these defects of character.
7. Humbly asked Him to remove our shortcomings.
8. Made a list of all persons we had harmed and became willing to make amends to all of them.
9. Made direct amends to such people wherever possible, except when doing so would injure them or others.
10. Continued to take personal inventory, and when we were wrong promptly admitted it.
11. Sought through prayer and meditation to improve our conscious contact with God as we understood Him, praying only for knowledge of His will for us and the power to carry that out.
12. Having had a spiritual awakening as the result of these steps, we tried to carry this message to alcoholics, and to practice these principles in all our affairs.

to God or a "higher power." But from the beginning, AA presented itself as open to (and effective for) religious and secular persons alike, with the definition of its spiritual component left to the participant.

The groups are self-organized, without oversight from a central office. There are no professionals in the system. Everyone who wishes can be partnered with a sponsor. The sponsor identifies as someone who has achieved some modicum of sobriety and has experience with the twelve steps. The sponsor, a volunteer who is not financially compensated, will meet with the participant throughout the process and is on call for emergencies.

AA is notable for elements that decidedly distinguished it from the medical approach to addiction. It is a peer-to-peer self-help organization. The qualifications of its leaders are that they should have experienced the same affliction and degradations shared by all its members. The program encourages participants to leave at the door of their meetings all the distinguishing features of status or background, using only first names, to maintain the anonymity headlined in the title. The proceedings of the group are supposed to be confidential. The leader of the meeting will often say, "What you hear in this meeting stays in this meeting." The participants chime in, "Here, here." It insists on approaching the addiction in the context of the whole person and all their relations, including their spiritual life, as a problem inextricable from that whole nexus.

The basic paradigm of the twelve steps clearly reflects a religious prototype: the Christian, and even specifically Protestant, path of salvation, with its elements of confession, repentance, and regeneration. The signature moment in an AA meeting comes when any member speaks and introduces themselves with the ritual preface, "I'm John, and I'm an alcoholic." To attend a meeting is already to take the major step of dispelling the characteristic layers of denial that prevent this acknowledgement. The acknowledgement stands as the hurdle at the door that prevents so many from entering, the base level qualification to be helped.

The parallel Protestant moment would be the confession that I am a sinner and unable to save myself. Only from this frank insight, and faith in the power of deliverance beyond my own, is reception of undeserved grace from a higher power possible. The new, redeemed life that follows is, in Luther's famous formulation, one in which a person is simultaneously both sinful (according to one's continuing inclinations) and justified (according to God's gracious acceptance).[6] It is a bedrock principle of AA that, however long one may remain "clean," without drinking, one does not stop being an alcoholic, someone who is powerless over liquor. The hope is to be, day by day, both sober and an alcoholic. In this respect, AA reflected a generic Protestant Christianity, stripped down and laser focused on a single form of human estrangement.

AA seeks to be a big tent on the spirituality dimension of recovery, but it has inspired variations specifically responsive to differences on this front. The obvious religious resonances of AA led some to seek an explicitly atheistic or agnostic alternative. Several such organizations have been formed, often in loose affiliation with AA, using a revised version of the twelve steps. They are linked within a network, S.O.S. (Secular Organizations for Sobriety). The initials are also used to stand for "save our selves," to indicate that the focus is not on divine help but individual responsibility.[7] Part of the concern expressed by these groups has to do with what they perceive as an element of humiliation or self-abasement required in a twelve step approach. "Hitting rock bottom," in terms of the disruption of one's personal life, is something AA members often report as the prelude to their true transformation. It is an observation, not a prescription. But alternative approaches fear that even to implicitly endorse the benefits of such an experience constitutes an abusive and unhealthy prescription for those who may already be devalued and powerless.

Over the past thirty years, a more explicitly Christian, biblically focused version of the twelve-step program has grown up, "Celebrate Recovery."[8] In their rubric, the basic anonymous self-identification is revised: "Hi, I'm Cathy. I seek to follow Jesus, and I struggle with alcohol." This identification avoids a permanent label of one's self as an alcoholic, an addict. Out of concerns that overlap with those of the secular programs, such an approach seeks to preserve respect for the agency and value of the person confronting their impairment. The participant *struggles* with addiction, but is not defined by her addiction. She stresses her identity as a spiritual being, as well as the

---

[6]See Martin Luther, "Preface to the Epistle of St. Paul to the Romans," in *Martin Luther, Selections from His Writings*, 1st ed., Anchor Books, A271, ed. Martin Luther and John Dillenberger (Garden City, NY: Doubleday, 1961), 19–34.
[7]Kelly Fitzgerald, "4 Ways Atheists and Agnostics Recover," *The Recovery Village*, https://www.therecoveryvillage.com/recovery/4-ways-atheists-agnostics-recover/#:~:text=AA%20Agnostica%20and%20Secular%20AA,key%20difference%20from%20traditional%20AA.
[8]Celebrate Recovery, "Celebrate Recovery," https://celebraterecovery.com.

specific power and model from whom she seeks support. This is not to say that a person who struggles with addiction may not relapse—even after several years. But, always to be defined by your addiction is harmful. A person is more than their illness, more than their addiction.

From a theological perspective, Christians have a multidimensional view of human nature, rooted in the large scope of salvation history. We have a created nature ("made in the image of God") whose primordial character is never effaced. We are also fallen, broken creatures, whose estrangement from God and neighbor twists all of our capacities, a little or a lot. Yet ours is also the humanity God has assumed in the incarnation of Christ, whose relation with God we can participate in, healing sin and uplifting our distinctive personalities. Finally, we have an eschatological destiny, in which our created being will be perfected in communion with God and other creatures. Luther's "at the same time justified and yet sinners" is a lot to hold together, but it is, at best, an abbreviation. It is all of these reference points that combine in a kind of symphonic unity to frame our "nature." We are, all at the same time, created in the image of God, fallen into estrangement and bondage, savingly infused with new life and agency, and finally fulfilled through hope.

To know which of these receives relative emphasis, we ask "what time is it?"—not only what time in the history of salvation, which provides the pattern of the four reference points, but in any individual life journey. For many people struggling with addiction, it is indeed time to stress the aspects that AA chose to emphasize: brokenness, loss of control, turning outward for help, repentance and rebuilding relationships.

Those who undergo addiction, and their loved ones and caregivers, often evoke a spiritual or religious dimension to the experience. This is particularly true in relation to the all-consuming and transforming power of the attraction to the addictive substance. Heroin becomes a god, an extremely jealous god, demanding everything in one's life be subjugated to its power. The substance or the activity delivers a moment of bliss, and offers repetition of the same, on the condition that you sacrifice your relationships, your future, your financial and physical well-being. If you take that bag of heroin, snort it, smoke it, or inject it, for that ten dollars all of your problems go far, far away.[9]

---

[9] At the time of writing, heroin in New Haven, Connecticut costs about ten dollars per bag. Ten bags make a bundle, which can be purchased at a discount of around 60 dollars. Such information may

This is a bargain, or appears so, the more distressing the conditions of your daily life. Your lousy job, gone. Your busted-up relationship, gone. That horrible trauma from your childhood, gone. That nagging guilt from the mistake you made, gone. Completely gone. Drugs work. A bag of heroin is good for about an hour or two. To live your life completely in a state of altered consciousness, you need about ten bags of heroin a day.

The problem with drugs is that you lose not only your problems, you lose yourself. The drug that was your escape from your problems becomes the problem itself. You lose your life to the drug, and the drug becomes your life. And suddenly, every fiber of your being, every waking moment, focuses on getting the next hit. The person addicted will do anything—sell her mom's jewels, steal, prostitute. But, in becoming self-absorbed, the one addicted loses herself. The drug becomes an insatiable false god whose demands never cease.

Liberation from such a consuming power often requires the assistance of an equally demanding one. It is no surprise that aspects of more conservative or evangelical Christian theologies, or of correlatives in other religious traditions, are prominent in recovery movements, especially among those without the resources to access costlier rehabilitation programs. It is not only the level of power attributed to the divine that is in play, but the higher demand (in terms of time, religious community engagement, and scope of the areas of life that are managed on religious terms) of membership in such groups that provides a counterweight to the addiction. If every waking moment is haunted by the thought of and the opportunity for getting high, then it is a feature and not a bug to have a religious script that not only helps fill that time, but also orders it in terms of activities like prayer, Bible reading, and group involvement and accountability.

Medical Models

Since the rise of AA, the medical model has changed dramatically. It came to regard addiction as a genuine disease, rooted in genetics and brain chemistry. For this disease, there were, for the first time, medications that could intervene in the chemical and neurological patterns associated with

---

not be taught in medical school, but it is an important indicator for those treating addiction.

substance abuse. The pharmacological model was supplemented with an updated psychological model, where cognitive behavioral therapy is employed to identify triggers driving the abuse and to manage stress. Under the care of a physician, a patient can be placed on a long-term opioid such as methadone or a blocker such as naltrexone that blunts the effect of drugs when taken. Ever so slowly, over weeks to months or even years, the dose is lowered so that the patient does not suffer withdrawal.

There are great benefits to the new medical model. Perhaps the most important is that it lifts much of the shame and stigma from the condition of addiction. Addiction can be considered in major part a medical disease with a medical treatment, not a fault or even a crime to be attributed simply to the patient's bad choices. Like eczema or hypertension, addiction requires diagnosis and care. This can provide enormous relief to a patient and can encourage them to acknowledge their situation and seek help. Unfortunately, this approach alone is not so effective: many will relapse and many will stay on chronic opioids for years.

The weakness in the medical model seems to correspond to some strengths in the spiritual model of addiction. A doctor can give a drug, like buprenorphine, to plug opioid receptors and thus dull the physiological cravings of addiction. But, in Ben's practice treating such persons over may years, he has rarely seen long term recovery or sobriety without some form of conversion, the *metanoia* or "turning around" from an old life to a new one. Medication can loosen the hold of the substance, but it cannot provide something of countervailing attraction, drawing one toward new satisfactions, relationships and habits. If addiction is viewed only as a biochemical process with a strong genetic component, do we run the risk of dismissing the person's role in their addiction? This could undervalue the importance of living out good choices in their recovery, particularly of finding a new orientation whose attractions go beyond canceling the pull of addiction.

Very few people dealing with addiction fail to see the negatives attached to it. In the twelve-step program, participants will say that addiction leads to "jail, institutions, or death." A patient of Ben's said to him, "I did not always get into trouble doing drugs, but when I did get into trouble, it was always because I did drugs." But to desire not to do drugs is not the same thing as effectively desiring something other than drugs. And the reformation of desire is one of the central themes of religious practice.

Addiction highlights the way in which the interpretive frameworks for religious and medical care are sometimes hard to disentangle from one another. Some conditions, medical or human, are extremely difficult to treat effectively. Addiction is probably at the top of that list. In this respect, the most powerful therapeutics we have are probably preventive ones, that may not look medical at all. In the chapter on religion and health data we saw the strong association of religious observance with improved all cause mortality. One pathway for that effect is certainly the protective effect of religious practice in lessening the frequency with which adherents acquire health-degrading conditions like addiction.[10]

We saw that although religious observance statistically correlates with improved mortality results, there are still areas where religious practice (or certain kinds of religious practice) correlate with more negative outcomes. There are religiously induced health problems, mental and otherwise. These are distinct from the situations we have described where religious faith may explicitly and consciously sacrifice better physical well-being in the service of some other end, such as care for others or solidarity against injustice. For instance, religious traditions and structures can be organized to rationalize behavior (sexual abuse of adherents by leaders, pre-existing mental illness in adherents, stigmatizing attitudes toward others). If there is power in religion and spirituality that can be deployed for healing, it is equally true that that power can become destructive.

Likewise, health damage may result from medical treatment: the hospital-acquired infection, the disease produced as a side effect of treatment, the damage from a medical mistake or misdiagnosis, the allergic reaction to a medication. In recent decades we saw a prime example of this in the field of addiction. Many doctors and patients shared a concern that the pain suffered by patients was not adequately appreciated or addressed by most physicians. The concern was that doctors under-diagnosed and under-treated pain.

The prescription was that they should be more aggressive in recognizing and medicating it. The pain charts that have become familiar to us all—the faces marked from one to ten—were products of a movement to take pain seriously and treat it as a vital sign in its own right. The preferred instruments for treating this pain, now being more readily diagnosed, were powerful analgesics of relatively recent development. These were ready at hand, aggressively marketed by the pharmaceutical companies that sold them.

---

[10]Brian J. Grim and Melissa E. Grim, "Belief, Behavior, and Belonging: How Faith Is Indispensable in Preventing and Recovering from Substance Abuse," *Journal of Religion and Health* 58, no. 5 (2019): 1713–52.

Opioids are extremely effective at treating pain, mood disorders, and anxiety ... in the short term.

This expanded the realm of addiction to include those whose initial dealers were not street sellers of illicit drugs, but trusted physicians writing prescriptions for recovery from surgery, chronic back pain, orthopedic injuries, or treatment of bipolar disorder and depression. Though these medications quickly became part of the normal standard of care, some patients were at much greater risk from them than others because of a strong genetic predisposition, or the stresses of particular life circumstances, or simply because the drugs were more powerful than initially understood.

The resulting opioid epidemic represents a "perfect storm" that combined this new entry path toward addiction with the appearance of novel synthetic opioids such as fentanyl and carfentanil, which are hundreds of times more powerful by weight than previously known drugs like morphine.[11] Even small amounts of carfentanil absorbed through the skin can cause respiratory depression. When opioids are cut with carfentanil and other derivatives, the effect is devastating.

There are three main issues with opioids. First, ever-increasing doses are required to achieve the same effect in pain relief. This can happen quite rapidly over days to weeks. The oxycodone 5 mg tab that worked for that ankle fracture in the beginning no longer is effective. 10 mg, then 20 mg, then 30 mg is required. The second issue with opioid addiction is the withdrawal. If opioids make a person feel calm, blissful, and pain-free, withdrawal makes a person feel anxious, miserable, and hypersensitive. Withdrawal starts with the creepy crawlies—formication is the medical term from *formica* which means ant in Latin. The third concern has to do with inadvertent exposure. Street drugs of all sorts often have been laced with these powerful synthetic opioids, heightening the danger for existing users of heroin or even marijuana.

The widening net of exposure to these drugs, combined with their elevated potency, meant that both addiction and fatal overdoses increased. The impact of this touches nearly every corner of society and destroys lives, families, and communities. In the United States, more than three million people are addicted to opioids with 500,000 of those addicted to heroin. Nearly a third of the United States population is either struggling with

---

[11] For an account of the opioid epidemic, see Patrick Radden Keefe, *Empire of Pain: The Secret History of the Sackler Dynasty*, 1st ed. (New York: Doubleday, 2021).

addiction or has had a family member struggle.[12] This means that if you or your family have not been touched by opioid addiction, then one of your neighbors has.

There are unscrupulous practitioners in both religion and medicine, but few doctors who prescribed opioids were trying to make patients addicted. They were conscientiously treating pain. However, they were, in the long run, practicing reductionistic medicine in that they treated the pain but not the suffering. They kept writing prescriptions, oblivious to the new disease they were feeding. Or, as the patients moved from their medical opioids to street versions, doctors failed to recognize the epidemic of "deaths of despair" that now followed. People who had fallen into addiction by a medical route, found that the competing "jealous gods" that might have helped pull them away (employment, family connections, community organizations, churches) were at the same time undermined. Religious leaders and communities, dealing with the fallout of addiction, tended to focus on emergency treatment for those suffering, but have little bandwidth or perspective to engage with medical providers to reshape the treatments that fueled the problem.

Forgiveness as a Health Issue

An important feature of addiction recovery is forgiveness, a cornerstone in many religious frameworks, but rarely discussed in medicine. Forgiveness specifies an important portion of what is included in the spiritual program of AA. Many of the twelve steps bear directly on this topic: confessing to God and to others wrongs that we have done, seeking to make direct amends to people we have harmed, and seeking to improve our conscious contact with God. Although the word is not used explicitly, all of these steps appear proactively oriented toward the possibility of forgiveness for the addicted person, forgiveness from God and from those the addict has harmed. The first concrete steps are not to ask for forgiveness but to manifest repentance and care for those who have been harmed. We could also say that these activities lay a foundation for overcoming shame and self-loathing, for

---

[12] https://www.ncbi.nlm.nih.gov/books/NBK448203/#:~:text=Three%20million%20US%20citizens%20and,in%20a%20year%20time%20period.

growing the capacity to accept grace from God and from others, for self-forgiveness.

A number of recent studies have addressed this interface of religion and public health, some of them, notably, conducted under the umbrella of the Human Flourishing Program in the Department of Epidemiology at Harvard's Chan School of Public Health. A review of relevant studies, many of which controlled extensively for confounding variables, has indicated consistent evidence for a positive effect of forgiveness on depression, anxiety, and hope.[13] Clearly, this is a complex phenomenon. The concept of forgiveness is subject to careful analysis and distinctions in religious terms, and medical studies have tested it under varied definitions: forgiveness of others, self-forgiveness, divine forgiveness. One of these studies concluded "All forgiveness measures were positively associated with all psychosocial well-being outcomes, and inversely associated with depressive and anxiety symptoms."[14] A meta-analysis of studies bearing on physical health outcomes also found positive relations.[15]

Recently, the Harvard Human Flourishing Program organized the largest randomized cross-cultural interventional forgiveness study yet attempted.[16] The intervention that was administered was the brief (two week) self-directed use of a forgiveness workbook. Some 4,500 participants took part from around the world, in Colombia, Hong Kong, Indonesia, South Africa, and Ukraine. Its results verified that the general relation with positive mental health effects held in these cross-cultural contexts (chosen specifically for the existence of significant conflict as a background in the societies). A simple intervention in education and training in forgiveness produced measurable effects in the participants. One of the features of such a project is that it suggests that religiously derived insights and practices may be instructive for the development of public health measures that can be

---

[13] Loren Toussaint, David R. Williams, and Everett Worthington, *Forgiveness and Health: Scientific Evidence and Theories Relating Forgiveness to Better Health* (Dordrecht: Springer Netherlands; Imprint: Springer, 2015), doi:10.1007/978-94-017-9993-5.

[14] Ying Chen et al., "Religiously or Spiritually-Motivated Forgiveness and Subsequent Health and Well-Being among Young Adults: An Outcome-Wide Analysis," *The Journal of Positive Psychology* 14, no. 5 (2019): 649.

[15] Yu-Rim Lee and Robert D. Enright, "A Meta-Analysis of the Association between Forgiveness of Others and Physical Health," *Psychology and Health* 34, no. 5 (2019): 626–43.

[16] See Shine Ho et al., *International Reach Forgiveness Intervention: A Multi-Site Randomized Controlled Trial* (2023), doi:10.31219/osf.io/8qzgw. And see the results from a specific site here: Andrea Ortega Bechara et al., "Do Forgiveness Campaign Activities Improve Forgiveness, Mental Health, and Flourishing?," *International Journal of Public Health* 69, no. 7 March (2024): 1605341.

effectively applied in a non-sectarian manner. In these studies, the effect of the short term forgiveness intervention on depression and anxiety was roughly equivalent to that demonstrated by more intensive existing therapies and treatments.

We are increasingly aware of forces with profound effects on mental and physical health that operate in social space: social media, loneliness, the decline in mediating institutions. We are, in many respects, under dystopic "treatments," whether this involves over-medication, algorithmically accelerated negative rumination in the online world, pandemic-enforced deficits in socialization. A positive appreciation for spiritual resources and the inclusion of such resources in public health approaches can perhaps offer some countervailing supports.

Professor Martha Minow, from Harvard Law School, reported that when her interest in forgiveness led her to the law school library, she found virtually no resources. Her visit to the university library yielded little more. Only when she turned to the divinity school library did she find relevant material that eventually led to her book, *When Should Law Forgive?*[17] Considerations of the type she investigated are what has led thirty-six states in the United States to enact laws that provide for medical practitioners to say "I'm sorry" to patients without having this turning automatically into legal liability. The space for simple confession and possible forgiveness is not only crucial for personal well-being. It can be a necessary condition for systems to practice self-criticism and reform.

Recent attention to forgiveness in the medical arena has focused almost exclusively on interpersonal forgiveness and self-forgiveness. This is understandable, though also ironic, since, for the vast majority of the world's religious population (contemporary and historical), forgiveness has been explicitly linked with a divine referent. Some scholars have begun to address that gap.[18] One early finding suggests that the experience of divine forgiveness precedes increases in interpersonal forgiveness. Being forgiven by God impels one to be more forgiving of others, rather than the other way around (forgiveness, or the lack of it, from other people determining how we will perceive God's action).[19]

---

[17] Martha Minow, *When Should Law Forgive?* (New York: W. W. Norton & Company, 2019).
[18] Frank D. Fincham, "Towards a Psychology of Divine Forgiveness," *Psychology of Religion and Spirituality* 14, no. 4 (2022): 451–61.
[19] Frank D. Fincham and Ross W. May, "Divine Forgiveness and Interpersonal Forgiveness: Which Comes First?" *Psychology of Religion and Spirituality* 15, no. 2 (2023): 167–73.

Addiction harms many more than those who are addicted. The knowledge of the pain visited on loved ones and friends is part of the suffering that goes with addiction. Some resolution or reconciliation for those losses is a big part of enabling people to get to new life on the other side.

Medicine and religion are natural allies in responding to addiction. If we treat addiction on a medical disease model, concerned with which cell receptors to block with medication, we offer significant practical assistance in mitigating cravings. We remove some of the stigma and shame of the condition. We do not account for the complexity of the whole person, and do little to offer sources of meaning and satisfaction in life to compete with the power of the substance being abused. A religious or spiritual approach emphasizes exactly such alternative constructive powers, and directly addresses the web of broken relationships that also need restoration. Faith offers an alternative ground for self-worth, while an addicted person struggles with repeated disappointments. Principles of forgiveness and reconciliation model hope to those longing for new life. The fullest spectrum of medical and spiritual treatments, appropriate to any given individual, offers the most promise.

References

Bechara, Andrea Ortega, et al. "Do Forgiveness Campaign Activities Improve Forgiveness, Mental Health, and Flourishing?" *International Journal of Public Health* 69, no. 7 (2024): 1605341.

Chen, Ying, Sion Kim Harris, Everett L. Worthington, and Tyler J. VanderWeele. "Religiously or Spiritually-Motivated Forgiveness and Subsequent Health and Well-Being among Young Adults: An Outcome-Wide Analysis." *The Journal of Positive Psychology* 14, no. 5 (2019): 649–58.

Cottam, S., S.N. Paul, O.J. Doughty, L. Carpenter, A. Al-Mousawi, S. Karvounis, and D.J. Done. "Does Religious Belief Enable Positive Interpretation of Auditory Hallucinations? A Comparison of Religious Voice Hearers with and without Psychosis." [In English]. *Cognitive Neuropsychiatry* 16, no. 5 (2011): 403–21.

Fincham, Frank D. "Towards a Psychology of Divine Forgiveness." *Psychology of Religion and Spirituality* 14, no. 4 (2022): 451–61.

Fincham, Frank D., and Ross W. May. "Divine Forgiveness and Interpersonal Forgiveness: Which Comes First?" [In English]. *Psychology of Religion and Spirituality* 15, no. 2 (2023): 167–73.

Fitzgerald, Kelly. "4 Ways Atheists and Agnostics Recover." *The Recovery Village*. https://www.therecoveryvillage.com/recovery/4-ways-atheists-agnostics-recover/#:~:text=AA%20Agnostica%20and%20Secular%20AA,key%20difference%20from%20traditional%20AA.

Grim, Brian J., and Melissa E. Grim. "Belief, Behavior, and Belonging: How Faith Is Indispensable in Preventing and Recovering from Substance Abuse." [In English]. *Journal of Religion and Health* 58, no. 5 (2019): 1713–52.

Ho, Shine, Everett Worthington, Richard Cowden, Andrea Bechara, Zhuo Chen, Elly Yuliandari, Shaun Joynt, et al. *International Reach Forgiveness Intervention: A Multi-Site Randomized Controlled Trial*. 2023. doi:10.31219/osf.io/8qzgw.

Keefe, Patrick Radden. *Empire of Pain: The Secret History of the Sackler Dynasty*. 1st ed. New York: Doubleday, 2021.

Lee, Yu-Rim, and Robert D. Enright. "A Meta-Analysis of the Association between Forgiveness of Others and Physical Health." *Psychology and Health* 34, no. 5 (2019): 626–43.

Luhrmann, Tanya M. *When God Talks Back: Understanding the American Evangelical Relationship with God*. 1st ed. New York: Alfred A. Knopf, 2012.

Luhrmann, Tanya M., Ben Alderson-Day, Ann Chen, Philip Corlett, Quinton Deeley, David Dupuis, Michael Lifshitz, et al. "Learning to Discern the Voices of Gods, Spirits, Tulpas, and the Dead." [In English]. *Schizophrenia Bulletin* 49, no. Supplement_1 (2023): S3–S12.

Luther, Martin, and John Dillenberger. *Martin Luther, Selections from His Writings*. Anchor Books, A271. 1st ed. Garden City, NY: Doubleday, 1961.

Minow, Martha. *When Should Law Forgive?* New York: W. W. Norton & Company, 2019.

Powers, Albert R., Claire Bien, and Philip R. Corlett. "Aligning Computational Psychiatry with the Hearing Voices Movement: Hearing Their Voices." [In English]. *JAMA Psychiatry (Chicago, Ill.)* 75, no. 6 (2018): 640–1.

Recovery, Celebrate. "Celebrate Recovery." https://celebraterecovery.com.

Toussaint, Loren, David R. Williams, and Everett Worthington. *Forgiveness and Health: Scientific Evidence and Theories Relating Forgiveness to Better Health*. Dordrecht: Springer, Netherlands: Imprint: Springer, 2015. doi:10.1007/978-94-017-9993-5.

10

Burnout as Spiritual Crisis

Chapter Outline

Burnout in Physicians and Clergy	184
Responses to Burnout	188
Burnout as Spiritual Crisis	190
Flourishing	192
A Way Forward	195

The first known literary reference to the word *burnout* is Graham Greene's novel, *The Burnt Out Case*. A London-based, high-end church architect experiences an episode of profound disengagement, and emotional fatigue. He flees his stable, upper-middle-class life and finds himself in central Africa, at a leprosarium run by the Catholic Church. In one passage, he compares himself to a leper:

> You heard what the doctor called me just now—one of the burnt-out cases. They are the lepers who lose everything that can be eaten away before they are cured... I've come to an end. This place, you might say, is the end. Neither the road, nor the river go any further.

And then, as if turning towards the reader, he asks, "You have been washed up here too, haven't you?"[1]

---

[1] Graham Greene, *A Burnt-out Case* (New York: Random House, 2010), 125.

Burnout in Physicians and Clergy

A burnt-out case of leprosy is a graphic image for a syndrome that describes half of all healthcare workers and perhaps one-third of clergy.[2] Addiction is an active disorder, its powerful gravity pulling someone away from all normal activities and their satisfactions. Burnout is a kind of blankness, a dull emptiness that spreads over the vocational world where one once found energy and purpose. It is a prime risk factor for addiction, since alcohol or a drug can become the means to get through an unrewarding work day, or to compensate for enjoyments one no longer finds there. The profound vocational character of medicine and ministry, which is to say the expectation that the work is intrinsically animated with a deep purpose, makes it initially surprising that burnout should be so widespread. Burnout is a condition that has less to do with physiology and more to do with the realm of meaning and community. It is a spiritual condition as much as a medical one, but it has enormous impact on our contemporary medical world.

Burnout was first described in the psychology literature by Christina Maslach in the 1970s as a way of understanding a constellation of job-related symptoms that well described Greene's architect.[3] Maslach found that people in public-facing, people-intensive jobs, such as teachers and social workers, were at risk of suffering from a cluster of symptoms: *emotional exhaustion, disengagement, and lack of purpose.*[4] The emotional exhaustion was not just the fatigue of a hard day's work, but rather the sense of being completely depleted of inner resources. The disengagement manifested as an apathy for the work, a calcified indifference towards the client. The grind of the job results in a lack of purpose, a sense of futility, a feeling that nothing one does makes a difference in the world.

---

[2] On physician burnout see Tait D. Shanafelt et al., "Changes in Burnout and Satisfaction with Work-Life Integration in Physicians and the General Us Working Population between 2011 and 2020," *Mayo Clinic Proceedings* 97, no. 3 (2022): 491–506. On clergy burnout, see Christopher J. Adams et al., "Clergy Burnout: A Comparison Study with Other Helping Professions," *Pastoral Psychology* 66, no. 2 (2017): 147–75; Benjamin R. Doolittle, "The Impact of Behaviors Upon Burnout among Parish-Based Clergy," *Journal of Religion and Health* 49, no. 1 (2010): 88–95.
[3] Christina Maslach, Susan E. Jackson, and Michael P. Leiter, *Maslach Burnout Inventory Manual*, 3rd ed. (Palo Alto, CA: Consulting Psychologists Press, 1996).
[4] Ibid.

Burnout is highly correlated with major depressive disorder, but is different in a few important ways.[5] Burnout is job related. If a nurse with burnout has a day off, he can still enjoy gardening, walk the dog, and spend time with the kids. Depression is characterized by a lack of pleasure and low energy across all life experiences, both at work and away from it. The three domains of burnout hang together, but not completely. It is possible to be emotionally exhausted but also have a high sense of personal accomplishment. Healthcare workers in the early months of the Covid pandemic described this.[6] Usually, though, emotional exhaustion, depersonalization, and lack of accomplishment reinforce each other, leading to a chronic, dispirited malaise.[7]

Burnout is widespread. In 2021, a study by the American Psychological Association among 1,501 US adult workers, across multiple professions, showed that 79 percent experienced work-related stress in the month prior to the survey.[8] 59 percent experienced negative consequences of work-related stress, lack of interest, motivation, or energy (26 percent) and lack of effort at work (19 percent). Another study by LinkedIn, the career networking site, among 16,000 US workers, showed that 41 percent met criteria for burnout, with the highest professions being project managers (50 percent), healthcare workers (49 percent), community and social services workers (48 percent), quality assurance officers (47 percent), and educators (45 percent).[9] Globally, the prevalence of burnout is 43 percent among healthcare workers and 41 percent among public health workers.[10,11] Among 10,000 workers,

---

[5] Irvin Sam Schonfeld and Renzo Bianchi, "Burnout and Depression: Two Entities or One?" *Journal of Clinical Psychology* 72, no. 1 (2016): 22–37.

[6] J. Hyman and B. Doolittle, "The Impact of the Covid-19 Pandemic on the Residency Experience: A Qualitative Study," *International Journal of Innovative Research in Medical Science* 8, no. 2 (2023): 58–63.

[7] Keri J.S. Brady et al., "Describing the Emotional Exhaustion, Depersonalization, and Low Personal Accomplishment Symptoms Associated with Maslach Burnout Inventory Subscale Scores in US Physicians: An Item Response Theory Analysis," *Journal of Patient-Reported Outcomes* 4, no. 1 (2020): 42.

[8] The American workforce faces compounding pressure, according to APA's 2021 Work and Well-being survey results. Accessed online on January 1, 2025, https://www.apa.org/pubs/reports/work-well-being/compounding-pressure-2021.

[9] LinkedIn Workforce Confidence Survey: Burnout is highest in these jobs. Accessed online on January 1, 2025, https://www.linkedin.com/news/story/burnout-is-highest-in-these-jobs-6873362/.

[10] R. Nagarajan et al., "Global Estimate of Burnout among the Public Health Workforce: A Systematic Review and Meta-Analysis," *Human Resources for Health* 22, no. 1 (2024): 30.

[11] A.R.M. Alanazy and A. Alruwaili, "The Global Prevalence and Associated Factors of Burnout among Emergency Department Healthcare Workers and the Impact of the Covid-19 Pandemic: A Systematic Review and Meta-Analysis," *Healthcare (Basel)* 11, no. 15 (2023): 2220.

across seven countries, the prevalence of burnout was 42 percent.[12] Graham Greene's spiritual leprosy in *The Burnt Out Case* has spread globally.

There is nothing dramatically special about doctors and ministers, then, in comparison with many other professions. The surprise comes from the assumption that they should be less liable to this particular problem, given the depth of vocational commitment involved and the meaningfulness of their work. It may also stem from our reluctance to consider that those who care for us could be impaired to be indifferent to our needs and less than diligent in their practice. Those served in medical and religious communities are heavily invested in the competence and faithfulness of practitioners that receive their trust.

Among healthcare workers, the prevalence of burnout has been unchanged for the past twenty years. Large cohort studies show the prevalence of burnout among physicians to be 45 to 55 percent.[13] The level of burnout amongst nurses, nurse practitioners, physician assistants and other members in the healthcare workforce are about the same.[14,15] While there is variability from year to year, with some fluctuations across specialties, burnout shows no sign of abating. Despite the increased awareness of mental health issues, the rise of Chief Wellness Officers, and the expansion of employee assistance programs, there has not been much improvement.

Burnout has serious downstream implications for all workers. The condition is associated with other mental health issues such as depression and addiction, as well as relationship stress and divorce.[16] Burnout has important implications in healthcare. It is estimated to cost the US healthcare

---

[12] Asana, Anatomy of Work Special Report. Accessed online on January 1, 2025, https://resources.asana.com/americas-anatomy-of-work-burnout-ebook.html.

[13] Tait D. Shanafelt, Omar Hasan, and Lotte N. Dyrbye, "Changes in Burnout and Satisfaction with Work-Life Balance in Physicians and the General Us Working Population between 2011 and 2014 (Vol 90, Pg 1600, 2015)," *Mayo Clinic Proceedings* 91, no. 2 (2016): 276.

[14] Tiffany Woo et al., "Global Prevalence of Burnout Symptoms among Nurses: A Systematic Review and Meta-Analysis," *Journal of Psychiatric Research* 123 (2020): 9–20.

[15] Timothy Hoff, Shannon Carabetta, and Grace E. Collinson, "Satisfaction, Burnout, and Turnover among Nurse Practitioners and Physician Assistants: A Review of the Empirical Literature," *Medical Care Research and Review* 76, no. 1 (2017): 3–31.

[16] Stephen D. Brown, Marilyn J. Goske, and Craig M. Johnson, "Beyond Substance Abuse: Stress, Burnout, and Depression as Causes of Physician Impairment and Disruptive Behavior," *Journal of the American College of Radiology* 6, no. 7 (2009): 479–85. Anik Debrot et al., "Daily Work Stress and Relationship Satisfaction: Detachment Affects Romantic Couples' Interaction Quality," *Journal of Happiness Studies* 19 (2018): 2283–301.

system $4.6 billion/year.[17] Physicians with burnout are more likely to commit errors and get sued.[18] For institutions, these errors result in a host of further issues. They can lead to patients needing to return to the hospital, visits for which insurance is less likely to pay. Even apart from identifiable doctor error, the patients of burned out doctors simply do not do as well as others.[19] If we think back to our discussion of the meaning response in Chapter Four, one can understand that patients who sense the disengagement and emotional exhaustion of their care giver would be negatively affected. A physician with burnout is more likely to leave their job. The cost of replacing that physician is two to three times the physician's annual salary in lost revenue, recruitment costs, and on-boarding.[20]

We are even burned out in responding to questions about burnout! Survey response rates are extremely low, often 6–8 percent.[21] This may be because people have become dubious that the information will make much difference, a perception that can only foster disengagement and pessimism. Annual engagement surveys from hospital systems and church adjudicatory bodies do not result in much action.

Clergy and chaplains tend to experience burnout at levels similar to those of other service-oriented professions, such as social workers, counselors, and teachers, with a prevalence around 30–35 percent.[22] This is somewhat lower than the level among healthcare workers. Clergy and chaplains have demanding, complex jobs. Typically they receive lower salaries than healthcare workers and, increasingly, they have lower social status. So it is somewhat surprising that their prevalence of burnout tends to be lower than

---

[17]Shasha Han et al., "Estimating the Attributable Cost of Physician Burnout in the United States," *Annals of Internal Medicine* 170, no. 11 (2019): 784–90.
[18]Chris J. Li et al., "Physician Burnout and Medical Errors: Exploring the Relationship, Cost, and Solutions," *American Journal of Medical Quality* 38, no. 4 (2023): 196–202.
[19]E. S. Williams et al., "The Relationship of Organizational Culture, Stress, Satisfaction, and Burnout with Physician-Reported Error and Suboptimal Patient Care: Results from the Memo Study," *Health Care Manage Rev.* 32, no. 3 (2007): 203–12.
[20]Tait Shanafelt, Joel Goh, and Christine Sinsky, "The Business Case for Investing in Physician Well-Being," *JAMA Internal Medicine* 177, no. 12 (2017): 1826–32.
[21]Shanafelt, Hasan, and Dyrbye, "Changes in Burnout and Satisfaction with Work-Life Balance in Physicians and the General Us Working Population between 2011 and 2014 (Vol 90, Pg 1600, 2015)." Longitudinal intervention trials are often small and of short duration. While careful analysis is done to try to assure that respondents reflect the larger physician population, this is still an inference. We are really not sure about the true prevalence of burnout among physicians, but there is no doubt that it is significant
[22]Adams et al., "Clergy Burnout: A Comparison Study with Other Helping Professions." Doolittle, "The Impact of Behaviors Upon Burnout among Parish-Based Clergy."

global averages. This may be due to the mission-driven focus of clergy: a strong sense of vocation that from the beginning "prices in" many of the sacrifices associated with the work.[23] It may be that clergy have higher levels of communal support, for they often work in the midst of congregations, with regular schedules of worship and interpersonal activities. There may be a kind of protective balance in the work of many clergy, which involves a steady round of celebratory liturgical and personal events (like weddings and baptisms) alongside stressful crises and tragedies. There may be a selection bias: those electing to become clergy may simply more often have personality traits supporting optimism or resilience than those in other demanding jobs. But the difference is only a relative one. Burnout is certainly serious among clergy and chaplains, with a significant impact in terms of people leaving the vocation and experiencing mental health issues. The features and symptoms of clergy and chaplain burnout are similar to the chronic burnout experienced by so many in modern society.

Responses to Burnout

Burnout for many years was placed at the feet of those suffering from it, the healthcare workers or religious leaders. They were not meditating enough, not exercising enough, not enjoying the kids' sports games enough. Burnout was their fault. Through proper training, burnout could be ameliorated. This fix-it-through-training model is a popular motif in medical education. We identify a problem, design a curriculum, administer the training to the appropriate subjects, and the problem is solved. For years, national medical education meetings would offer workshops on self care: resilience, mindfulness, and well-being. Religious institutions, like denominations, offered very similar programs, though these always included a category of spiritual care: deepening prayer and devotional life. None of these workshops seemed to make much overall difference.

More recently, hospital leaders have realized that the individual might not be to blame, but rather systemic issues might be at play. Burnout might be an appropriate response to a toxic situation. The cause might be long working

---

[23] B.R. Doolittle, "Burnout and Coping Among Parish-based Clergy," *Mental Health, Religion & Culture* 10, no. 1 (2007): 31–8.

hours, with minimal support, and impossible demands. Hospital systems administered well-being surveys, hired Chief Wellness Officers, and expanded employee assistance programs. Physician well-being is now touted as the fourth pillar of healthcare, along with improved care quality, improved patient experience, and improved cost.[24] And yet there has been no improvement in physician well-being. Why?

Several forces are at play. First, efforts by institutions to change the work environment have been largely superficial. The work demands are great. There are not enough nurses to fill the shifts, not enough doctors for the offices and wards. Expanded employee assistance programs are important for when things get really tough, like in the case of mental illness or the need for family medical leave. But this does not change the day-in, day-out grind of the night shift. Chief wellness officers offer a prophetic voice, championing well-being. But by themselves they cannot change culture or systems. That requires a more drastic overhaul in the work environment: more job sharing, fewer hours, more ancillary help. All this costs money, and the system is not ready to pay.

Second, intrinsic forces contribute to continuing burnout. Physicians tend to be driven people, with a note of perfectionism—and maybe some ego—thrown in. They studied hard to get into medical school and hunkered down through residency, often deferring marriage and family, with the vague expectation that things would be better after residency. They were not. Healthcare workers are also service-oriented. They are people-pleasers. The motivations behind their choice of career are complicated—intellectual challenge, social prestige, altruism, and a decent salary—but they tended to assume that after their long training job satisfaction would be assured.

One physician captured this sentiment in a Canadian well-being study:

> I believe that most physicians unconsciously contracted with society to pursue their profession to the utmost of their ability and energy, to keep up their skills, and do whatever was needed to promote patient care. In return we expected respect, the equipment to do the job, and freedom from financial anxieties. All three of these expectations have been abrogated, yet we continue to fulfill our side of the contract in confusion, disbelief, and a sense of betrayal.[25]

---

[24]Thomas M.D. Bodenheimer and Christine M.D. Sinsky, "From Triple to Quadruple Aim: Care of the Patient Requires Care of the Provider," *Annals of Family Medicine* 12, no. 6 (2014): 573–6.
[25]P. Sullivan and L. Buske, "Results from Cma's Huge 1998 Physician Survey Point to a Dispirited Profession," *Canadian Medical Association Journal (CMAJ)* 159, no. 5 (1998): 525.

Burnout as Spiritual Crisis

Burnout looks much more like a spiritual crisis than a medical one, even though we do not usually frame it that way. This is not to suppose that it is a purely individual matter, as assumed in the workshop approach discussed earlier, to be solved in some kind of contemplative solitude. The numb disengagement we are discussing need not only manifest itself in our work lives. Many testify to something similar in terms of their response to injustice and suffering on a larger, social level. In fact, burnout in health and religious workers is notable because of its deep overlap with this dynamic, since the jobs of these workers entail a daily encounter with the individual, human faces of those wider forces of disruption and destruction. People entered these professions, often, with the intention and expectation that they would, in some concrete way, respond to the total sum of human suffering, pain, and injustice. The inability to see or trust that this connection exists in their daily activities is one of the factors that lead to burnout.

As one reads accounts of burnout, it is hard not to be reminded of the kind of diagnosis for the general human condition we have earlier referred to in twentieth-century existentialist writers. In Samuel Beckett's play, *Waiting for Godot*, the two main characters are waiting, waiting, waiting for a man, Godot, to appear. They do not know him. They have never met him. They do not know why they are waiting for him. And yet, they wait. Their waiting is futile, for Godot never appears. They consider suicide. Estragon, one of the main characters, exclaims, "Nothing happens. Nobody comes, nobody goes. It's awful."[26] This dark parable suggests that such chronic, nagging futility is all there is to life. In some ways, this outlook seems more like clinical depression, as described earlier, than burnout. But for religious workers and healthcare workers, the sense of general life meaning and purpose is often deeply implicated in their work, and it is hard to limit burnout to a "9-5" question. When people's experience of their daily work, a work that places them in intimate contact with human illness and suffering, begins to take on a *Godot* quality—"Nothing happens, Nothing changes"— that experience rarely remains compartmentalized. Suicide levels for health

---

[26]Samuel Beckett, *Waiting for Godot: A Tragicomedy in Two Acts* (London: Faber and Faber, 1956), 34.

care workers are found to be high relative to other similarly educated professionals.[27]

An existential crisis occurs when there is a gap between one's self-perceived identity and their lived reality. A nurse may enter the profession with a strong desire to relieve the suffering of vulnerable patients. The reality she encounters instead is the burden of endless charting and time-consuming protocols. A physician may believe that the doctor's role is to find the clues that lead to a diagnosis, counsel the patient through difficult decisions, and then administer a salvific treatment. The reality may be a life burdened by administrative tasks mandated by insurance companies and demanded by electronic medical record keeping. The result of this existential crisis is one of drifting purposelessness. What is the point?

Clergy experience parallel forms of burnout, and for many similar reasons: long hours, emotional stress from dealing with extreme human need, and high expectations. But there are factors particular to their vocation. Pastors often function as a "24 hour ER," a first line resort for crises of all sorts—financial, familial, medical. Unlike physicians, they cannot take refuge in a specialty which gives them a sense of control and competence, and defer all other problems to some other provider. Religious leaders often feel the pressure of expectations to be exemplary moral and spiritual examples. For this reason, it may be hard for them to acknowledge difficulties or to seek help, including medical help. They also often become lightning rods for conflicts within their congregations or communities.

For a religious leader, it is unusual for a burnout issue related to work not to also become also a spiritual issue, since the job is so closely tied to faith, as the motivation that called a person into the vocation and as also the reference point of the work itself. One ironic benefit of this is that spiritual struggle is a recognized feature of religious life itself. Doubt, dry spells of spiritual practice, the need for renewal, are all things with which religious people are familiar and which are regularly addressed in corporate life. These resources are mismatched when one expects simply, say, to "pray away" a mental illness. But there are genuine protective resources in these traditions.

For a physician or nurse, "losing faith in medicine" may not be an experience with which they are familiar, for which they are prepared, or against which they have developed any protective resources. Medical

---

[27] F. Dutheil et al., "Suicide among Physicians and Health-Care Workers: A Systematic Review and Meta-Analysis," *PLoS One* 14, no. 12 (2019): e0226361.

education does not, for the most part, consider building capacities in students to sustain life in the medical field. There has been little research on the relationship between faith and burnout among physicians. What has been done indicates that an active spirituality corresponds to lower levels of burnout, but simple religious affiliation does not.[28]

Flourishing

Burnout is a term that comes from a disease model. It is a diagnosis. Medicine tends to focus on disease, rather than well-being. How do you fix burnout? But burnout is a kind of null set. It is what we see in the absence of something else: meaning, satisfaction, joy, purpose. People suffering burnout did not have an accident or acquire some random infection. They are missing something central to life, which appears in a medical model only as a byproduct. Rather than asking why we have become burned out, we can ask what well-being looks like. We can consider what it means to flourish, not just on a list of clinical measures (my body mass index, cholesterol levels, blood pressure) but in terms of what is missing in burnout.

Instead of measuring burnout, we can ask, who is thriving in medicine, and why? Surprisingly, there has been no well-described model for physician thriving. To investigate this, Ben and a group of residents and faculty decided to interview physicians who were satisfied with their lives, who were *not* burned out. The first group was comprised of primary care physicians, a specialty with a high prevalence of burnout.[29]

Physicians were keen to take part in the conversations. Ben and his colleagues focused on those who were at least in mid-career, physicians who had survived the rigors of the profession and were still going strong. They used validated questionnaires, developed by Maslach, to make sure that they were *not* burned out. They confirmed that they were satisfied with their career and their lives overall. They then asked open-ended questions about why they were satisfied with their career and their lives. They asked about job demands, finances, spirituality, exercise, family support. By asking open-

---

[28] I.O. Whitehead et al., "Systematic Review of the Relationship between Burnout and Spiritual Health in Doctors," *BMJ Open* 13, no. 8 (2023): e068402.
[29] Katherine Ann Gielissen et al., "Thriving among Primary Care Physicians: A Qualitative Study," *Journal of General Internal Medicine: JGIM* 36, no. 12 (2021): 3759–65.

ended questions that explored broad aspects of their lives, they sought wisdom that might be applicable to others.

Since that initial study, Ben and his colleagues have conducted interviews with more than 200 participants from different communities: resident physicians during a pandemic, physicians in Pakistan, palliative care workers in South Africa, people with paralysis who use wheelchairs. While there are some subtle differences between these disparate groups, there are also some strong shared signals.

First, thriving people all identified strong social connections. Some described a vast network of large families. One doctor said, "Every weekend, it seems I'm going to a baptism or a bar mitzvah or a wedding for someone in my family." Others describe overlapping smaller communities. One participant had to leave the interview early, "I'm in a bicycle club. We ride every week. I can't keep my guys waiting." One emergency physician explained, "Without the human touch, life has no meaning for me. Me being with a friend is soul food."

The importance of social connection does not seem to apply to extroverts only. Many physicians described smaller, meaningful relationships. One physician said, "I only have a few close friends, but they are the world to me." Many of the participants noted how important the social connections of a tight staff are for well-being. One participant said, "What helps me thrive... is my staff. I'm blessed with a great staff. We get along. We're like a big family, and that's what makes me happy to come to work."[30]

In fact, personality type is a complex construct. In the study of emergency physicians, thriving physicians tended to describe themselves as both introverted and extroverted. One physician said, "The introvert side of you gives you your intellectual and moral integrity while the extrovert side of you allows you to be a leader in the department. You need to be both really." Another said, "The introversion helps you to study and do well, and the extroversion helps you be good in a team." [31]

Second, thriving people have a sense of purpose. A physician who cares for children with HIV remarked about the importance of vocation. Being a physician and caring for the vulnerable is "knowing I am exactly where I am

---

[30]Ibid.
[31]Jesse Kase and Benjamin Doolittle, "Job and Life Satisfaction among Emergency Physicians: A Qualitative Study," *PloS One* 18, no. 2 (2023): e0279425-e25.

supposed to be."³² Intrinsic values rather than salary or social standing, is what gives the physicians meaning in their work. One primary doctor said, "I just think at that point I decided my life was going be about helping people. That I saw suffering that I could actually do something for. And that, I think, has informed my whole life."³³ Across all types of thriving physicians—emergency department physicians, primary care physicians, physicians from South African and Pakistan—they each articulated a sense of intrinsic vocation.

Interestingly, very few of these physicians spoke about maintaining work-life balance. Work-life balance is a buzzword in the well-being world. Appropriate boundaries are important, of course, but these thriving physicians did not discuss the importance of switching off their work to begin living. In fact, it was the opposite. One physician described being part of the board of directors of a summer camp. "Why?" I asked. "Were you the camp doctor? Did your kids go to the camp?" She explained that she believed it was her mission as a physician to care for children. Serving on a board was an important extension of her mission.

Many of these physicians explicitly mentioned religious or spiritual resources in their lives. For some, it showed up implicitly (their network of social support included family and friends, many of whom were embedded in religious communities). Many did not have any direct connection to religious organizations or practice. But their lives were marked by qualities that are more often talked about in spiritual than in medical terms.

Clearly, a religious commitment and community is one way that these qualities can be evoked and maintained. Ben and Mark are familiar with doctors who, with their families, banded together for some years to live as a small Christian community. The community included practicing physicians and those at various stages of medical education, all within the same wider medical network in their community. The purpose was to support each other in medical training and practice, both in practical ways related to the medicine and in spiritual ways related to their sense of vocation and mission ("everything else is hard"). It is not uncommon in major teaching hospitals now to see large numbers of Muslim staff members in the chapel together at a daily hour of prayer. These are ways of explicitly nurturing some of the

---

³²Annemarie E. Oberholzer and Benjamin R. Doolittle, "Flourishing, Religion, and Burnout among Caregivers Working in Pediatric Palliative Care," *International Journal of Psychiatry in Medicine* 59, no. 6 (2024): 727–39.
³³Gielissen et al., "Thriving among Primary Care Physicians: A Qualitative Study."

elements of flourishing Ben and his fellow researchers identified. Strong social connections, purpose, a happy blending of work and life—these things exist in many forms. But they also come in spiritual packages, belonging to particular religious traditions or derived from them. One of the benefits of the packages is that they were not conceived with the narrow aim of providing a meaningful life as a medical professional in our contemporary environment. They are aiming at a vision of human flourishing more comprehensive than that. But it still comes with the package.

As we said earlier, this is not to commend some retreat to a private spirituality. It is precisely the social connections and the sense of purpose that are part of this flourishing life that empower people and groups to change institutions or model new ways of doing things. One of Ben's speaking engagements took him to the School of Medicine at Loma Linda University in California, an institution of the Seventh Day Adventist Church. The mission of the School of Medicine is "to continue the teaching and healing ministry of Jesus Christ as we educate future medical professionals to excel in their chosen field."[34] The school provides an excellent medical education by the usual accreditation standards. But it also has long been on the leading edge of aspects of medicine that only recently have become widely appreciated—such as nutrition and life style—while maintaining a deep connection between religious care, including prayer, and medical care. It is a cardinal principle of its medical education that its students should be equipped to flourish in the integration of their faith with their vocation, as well as to heal others.

A Way Forward

After dozens of interviews with thriving physicians from around the world, Ben began to see themes emerging that he could share in medical education. The other major tributary was a course that our colleague Miroslav Volf developed for Yale undergraduates. The course is called "Life Worth Living."[35] It is organized around the idea of flourishing. What does it mean for a

---

[34]See https://medicine.llu.edu.
[35]See the best-selling book that derived from the course. Miroslav Volf, Matthew Croasmun, and Ryan McAnnally-Linz, *Life Worth Living: A Guide to What Matters Most* (New York: The Open Field/Penguin Life, 2023).

human being to flourish? The great religious and philosophical traditions of the world have all had answers to that question: a Buddhist answer, a Stoic answer, a Jewish answer. The course simply asks students to consider: what is *their* answer? Ben adapted the course as a short term offering he could teach in the medical school.

Aristotle used a word, *eudaimonia*, variously translated as flourishing or thriving. The *eu-* prefix means "well" or "good," and *daimonia* means "spiritedness" or the divine power within. Eudaimonia, then, is "being of good spirit," which came to mean well-being, or happiness. This, according to Aristotle, was the goal of life. The crucial question was what constituted *eudaimonia*. Which really meant, what makes life worth living?

The Stoics contended that well-being equaled virtue. Live according to reason, justice, and duty, and one will be content in the greatest good, whatever circumstance befalls you. Marcus Aurelius, the consummate philosopher-king was a renowned Stoic. He wrote "Concentrate every minute . . . on doing what's in front of you with precise and genuine seriousness, tenderly, willingly, with justice. And on freeing yourself from all other distractions."[36] The Epicureans argued instead that *eudaimonia* was pleasure and that virtues served a flourishing life to the extent that they fostered that good. Pleasure is the content of happiness, and the maximization of pleasure requires the use of reason. Don't party so much you die young, and so miss out on pleasure you could otherwise have enjoyed! Aristotle had his own answer to the question, where the highest form both of virtue and pleasure was an intellectual one: knowing and understanding the truth. There was joy in the right and the true. So *Eudaimonia* includes happiness, as we would think of it, but also purpose and doing good in the world.

What is important for our purposes is not Aristotle's answer, but the question. Ben's course asked his medical students to consider it as a key to their future flourishing in medicine. It is less about work-life balance, a balance between work and play, than it is about a connection between what is most meaningful to you (makes life worth living) and the activities in your life. Ancient Greek philosophy, empirical research, and Christian theology all overlap in the same counsel: consider what makes life worth living. Philosophy and religion not only encourage the question, but offer answers.

---

[36]Marcus Aurelius, Meditations, Translated by Gregory Hays, The Modern Library, New York, II (5), 92

Ben's course invites his students to find an answer and to cultivate it, as one of the best protections against burnout.

Christian theology offers its own rich vision of human flourishing, many of whose themes resonate with the outcomes of the qualitative studies we have discussed. First, theology offers to secular medicine the conviction that we are made in the image of God. Your value is not in your social status, your net worth, your academic rank. Your value derives not from what you have done. Your value is in being beloved by God. This is a powerful claim. Many physicians in the studies spoke of the intrinsic value of patients. A wider religious framework helps to sustain such a perception when it is tested. In our contemporary world our self-esteem is derived from social media "likes," while in Christian theology, we are validated not from social validation but divine validation.

Second, theology offers a path toward restoration and forgiveness. The liturgy of many Christian traditions guides worshippers through an arc of confession and reconciliation. We approach God; we confess our brokenness, individually and corporately; we acknowledge God's forgiveness and love; and we emerge from worship renewed. These rituals offer restoration. The Eucharist sustains participants in receiving common elements made holy.

Medicine does not do forgiveness and reconciliation well. The stakes are high. The fear of lawsuits is real. Institutional scrutiny without the assurance of forgiveness can lead to a desire to hide errors. Perhaps the closest exercise to a sacrament in this world is the morbidity and mortality rounds. A physician presents a patient who experienced an unexpected poor outcome, giving the history of the illness, diagnostic procedures, and the therapeutic interventions, and then explaining where things went wrong. Sometimes the physician is directly responsible for the outcome. More often, there was a Swiss cheese-type, systemic failure, with many small errors compiling towards a bad outcome. This exercise is meant to root out errors, systemic or individual, in an effort to do better the next time. These conferences sometimes model a spirit of vulnerable confession. But there is no mechanism for true reconciliation. The team, the physician, is left with the guilt, the regret, of a suffering patient. Medicine lacks a mechanism of reconciliation that theology can offer. There are limits to direct application of the religious pattern in a secular medical context, though we saw in Chapter Nine that even legal approaches to medical issues can be informed by religious perspectives. And the individual well-being of medical workers can be enhanced when they have recourse to practices of spiritual renewal apart from their employment.

Third, the importance of social connection was a strong signal from our qualitative studies. Religious communities organically model many of the qualities described by thriving physicians: a purpose-driven vocation embedded in a rich community. In an increasingly lonely age, religious community provides social glue, restorative relationships, and a sense of purpose that many crave in healthcare. For some, spiritual engagement fills out what is lacking in their employment or in their care. For others, these supportive models can inspire echoes in secular settings. Perhaps the most powerful and easily replicable intervention to reduce burnout is simply to break bread together. Several studies have shown that a family-style meal, without agenda or formal program, is associated with lower burnout among participating physicians.[37]

Religious communities organize themselves for the purposes of spiritual formation, through direct teaching, ritual, relationships, aesthetics (including music and art). Every workplace has some of these same dimensions, ways in which it is, often inadvertently, shaping people's experiences and outlook. Burnout is a sign that this formation has, to some extent become counterproductive. As individuals, we need to cultivate intrinsic values and social networks to sustain us in our work. As part of a system, we need to foster a humane work climate that encourages, supports, and forgives. Simply recognizing that these needs are inseparable from spiritual sources of meaning and purpose will help us heal the malaise that can hollow out the most important components of our medical systems, the human ones.

References

Adams, Christopher J., Holly Hough, Rae Jean Proeschold-Bell, Jia Yao, and Melanie Kolkin. "Clergy Burnout: A Comparison Study with Other Helping Professions." [In English]. *Pastoral Psychology* 66, no. 2 (2017): 147–75.

Alanazy, A.R.M., and A. Alruwaili. "The Global Prevalence and Associated Factors of Burnout among Emergency Department Healthcare Workers and the Impact of the Covid-19 Pandemic: A Systematic Review and Meta-Analysis." [In English]. *Healthcare (Basel)* 11, no. 15 (2023): 2220.

---

[37] A. Iyinbor and B. Doolittle, "Fostering Eudaimonia, Joy, and Connection among Resident Physicians: A Pilot Study," *International Journal of Innovative Research in Medical Science* 8, no. 10 (2023): 443–5, https://doi.org/10.23958/ijirms/vol08-i10/1752.

Beckett, Samuel. *Waiting for Godot: A Tragicomedy in Two Acts*. London: Faber and Faber, 1956.
Bodenheimer, Thomas M.D., and Christine M.D. Sinsky. "From Triple to Quadruple Aim: Care of the Patient Requires Care of the Provider." [In English U6—ctx_ver=Z39.88-2004&ctx_enc=info%3Aofi%2Fenc%3AUTF-8&rfr_id=info%3Asid%2Fsummon.serialssolutions.com&rft_val_fmt=info%3Aofi%2Ffmt%3Akev%3Amtx%3Ajournal&rft.genre=article&rft.atitle=From+Triple+to+Quadruple+Aim%3A+Care+of+the+Patient+Requires+Care+of+the+Provider&rft.jtitle=Annals+of+family+medicine&rft.au=Bodenheimer%2C+Thomas%2C+MD&rft.au=Sinsky%2C+Christine%2C+MD&rft.date=2014-11-01&rft.issn=1544-1709&rft.volume=12&rft.issue=6&rft.spage=573&rft.epage=576&rft_id=info:doi/10.1370%2Fafm.1713&rft.externalDBID=ECK1-s2.0-S1544170914601220&rft.externalDocID=1_s2_0_S1544170914601220&paramdict=en-us U7—Journal Article]. *Annals of Family Medicine* 12, no. 6 (2014): 573–6.
Brady, Keri J.S., Pengsheng Ni, R. Christopher Sheldrick, Mickey T. Trockel, Tait D. Shanafelt, Susannah G. Rowe, Jeffrey I. Schneider, and Lewis E. Kazis. "Describing the Emotional Exhaustion, Depersonalization, and Low Personal Accomplishment Symptoms Associated with Maslach Burnout Inventory Subscale Scores in Us Physicians: An Item Response Theory Analysis." *Journal of Patient-Reported Outcomes* 4, no. 1 (2020): 42.
Brown, Stephen D., Marilyn J. Goske, and Craig M. Johnson. "Beyond Substance Abuse: Stress, Burnout, and Depression as Causes of Physician Impairment and Disruptive Behavior." *Journal of the American College of Radiology* 6, no. 7 (2009): 479–85.
Debrot, Anik, Sebastian Siegler, Petra Klumb, and Dominik Schoebi. "Daily Work Stress and Relationship Satisfaction: Detachment Affects Romantic Couples' Interactions Quality." *Journal of Happiness Studies* 19 (2018): 2283–301.
Doolittle, Benjamin R. "The Impact of Behaviors Upon Burnout among Parish-Based Clergy." [In English]. *Journal of Religion and Health* 49, no. 1 (2010): 88–95.
Dutheil, F., C. Aubert, B. Pereira, M. Dambrun, F. Moustafa, M. Mermillod, J.S. Baker, et al. "Suicide among Physicians and Health-Care Workers: A Systematic Review and Meta-Analysis." [In English]. *PLoS One* 14, no. 12 (2019): e0226361.
Gielissen, Katherine Ann, Emily Pinto Taylor, David Vermette, and Benjamin Doolittle. "Thriving among Primary Care Physicians: A Qualitative Study." [In English]. *Journal of General Internal Medicine: JGIM* 36, no. 12 (2021): 3759–65.
Greene, Graham. *A Burnt-out Case*. New York: Random House, 2010.

Han, Shasha, Tait D. Shanafelt, Christine A. Sinsky, Karim M. Awad, Liselotte N. Dyrbye, Lynne C. Fiscus, Mickey Trockel, and Joel Goh. "Estimating the Attributable Cost of Physician Burnout in the United States." [In English]. *Annals of Internal Medicine* 170, no. 11 (2019): 784–90.

Hoff, Timothy, Shannon Carabetta, and Grace E. Collinson. "Satisfaction, Burnout, and Turnover among Nurse Practitioners and Physician Assistants: A Review of the Empirical Literature." *Medical Care Research and Review* 76, no. 1 (2017): 3–31.

Hyman, J., and B. Doolittle. "The Impact of the Covid-19 Pandemic on the Residency Experience: A Qualitative Study." *International Journal of Innovative Research in Medical Science* 8, no. 2 (2023): 58–63.

Kase, Jesse, and Benjamin Doolittle. "Job and Life Satisfaction among Emergency Physicians: A Qualitative Study." [In English]. *PloS one* 18, no. 2 (2023): e0279425-e25.

Li, Chris J., Yash B. Shah, Erika D. Harness, Zachary N. Goldberg, and David B. Nash. "Physician Burnout and Medical Errors: Exploring the Relationship, Cost, and Solutions." [In English]. *American Journal of Medical Quality* 38, no. 4 (2023): 196–202.

Maslach, Christina, Susan E. Jackson, and Michael P. Leiter. *Maslach Burnout Inventory Manual.* 3rd ed. Palo Alto, CA: Consulting Psychologists Press, 1996.

Nagarajan, R., P. Ramachandran, R. Dilipkumar, and P. Kaur. "Global Estimate of Burnout among the Public Health Workforce: A Systematic Review and Meta-Analysis." [In English]. *Human Resources for Health* 22, no. 1 (2024): 30.

Oberholzer, Annemarie E., and Benjamin R. Doolittle. "Flourishing, Religion, and Burnout among Caregivers Working in Pediatric Palliative Care." [In English]. *International Journal of Psychiatry in Medicine* 59, no. 6 (2024): 727–39.

Schonfeld, Irvin Sam, and Renzo Bianchi. "Burnout and Depression: Two Entities or One?" [In English]. *Journal of Clinical Psychology* 72, no. 1 (2016): 22–37.

Shanafelt, Tait D., Joel Goh, and Christine Sinsky. "The Business Case for Investing in Physician Well-Being." [In English]. *JAMA Internal Medicine* 177, no. 12 (2017): 1826–32.

Shanafelt, Tait D., Omar Hasan, and Lotte N. Dyrbye. "Changes in Burnout and Satisfaction with Work-Life Balance in Physicians and the General Us Working Population between 2011 and 2014 (Vol 90, Pg 1600, 2015)." [In English]. *Mayo Clinic Proceedings* 91, no. 2 (2016): 276.

Shanafelt, Tait D., Colin P. West, Christine Sinsky, Mickey Trockel, Michael Tutty, Hanhan Wang, Lindsey E. Carlasare, and Lotte N. Dyrbye. "Changes in Burnout and Satisfaction with Work-Life Integration in Physicians and the General Us Working Population between 2011 and 2020." [In English]. *Mayo Clinic Proceedings* 97, no. 3 (2022): 491–506.

Sullivan, P., and L. Buske. "Results from Cma's Huge 1998 Physician Survey Point to a Dispirited Profession." [In English]. *Canadian Medical Association Journal (CMAJ)* 159, no. 5 (1998): 525–8.

Volf, Miroslav, Matthew Croasmun, and Ryan McAnnally-Linz. *Life Worth Living: A Guide to What Matters Most*. New York: The Open Field/Penguin Life, 2023.

Whitehead, I.O., S. Moffatt, S. Warwick, G.F. Spiers, T.P. Kunonga, E. Tang, and B. Hanratty. "Systematic Review of the Relationship between Burn-out and Spiritual Health in Doctors." [In English]. *BMJ Open* 13, no. 8 (2023): e068402.

Williams, E. S., L.B. Manwell, T.R. Konrad, and M. Linzer. "The Relationship of Organizational Culture, Stress, Satisfaction, and Burnout with Physician-Reported Error and Suboptimal Patient Care: Results from the Memo Study." [In English]. *Health Care Management Review* 32, no. 3 (2007): 203–12.

Woo, Tiffany, Roger Ho, Arthur Tang, and Wilson Tam. "Global Prevalence of Burnout Symptoms among Nurses: A Systematic Review and Meta-Analysis." *Journal of Psychiatric Research* 123 (2020): 9–20.

11

Cancer, Immortality, and Christology

The Theological Resonance of Henrietta Lacks

Chapter Outline

Questions at the Edge of Medicine and Theology	207
Christology and Henrietta Lacks	209
In Memory of Her	216

On January 29, 1951, Henrietta Lacks presented herself for the evaluation of a "knot in her uterus" to Johns Hopkins Hospital, the only hospital in the Baltimore area that then treated Black patients. She came as an uneducated Black woman, who had grown up in a cabin that once served as slave quarters, seeking medical care from a powerful White-dominated institution at the forefront of American medical science, in a city with a history of brutal racism. A biopsy revealed a cancerous mass on her cervix. She received radium tube implants, the standard treatment at the time. During these treatments, two tissue samples were taken—one healthy and the other cancerous—without her explicit permission. The cancerous cells were given to Dr. George Otto Gey, an oncologist and researcher. Eight months later she perished from her disease. A partial autopsy showed that her cancer had widely metastasized. She was thirty-one years old and left five children and a husband.[1]

Despite all scientific attempts, it had so far been impossible to keep human cell lines alive in laboratories for more than a short time. Amazingly, Lacks' cancer cells continued to replicate, far exceeding the viability of any prior specimen in this respect, and showing no signs of stopping. These cells, distinguished by their virtual immortality, launched a new age of medical experimentation. They were labeled *HeLa*, based on the first two letters of the patient's first and last name. They were quickly, informally distributed through the medical research community and played a central role in the creation of many now standard treatments and vaccines. Jonas Salk used *HeLa* cells to develop the polio vaccine.[2] *HeLa* cells have been used to understand the impact of x-rays upon human cells, develop cancer therapeutics, study aging, and explore the pathogenesis of infectious diseases such as HIV, salmonella, and tuberculosis.[3] Seven researchers have won the Nobel Prize based on work that depended on *HeLa* cells.[4] More than 60,000 scholarly papers have been published using them.[5]

HeLa cells were famous within the scientific community, if not in the wider world. The woman from whom they came was not known in either. This changed in 2010. Rebecca Skloot's book *The Immortal Life of Henrietta Lacks* brought to public awareness her story and her family's struggle to come to terms with that legacy. The book has been adopted widely for study in high schools, universities, and medical schools across the country. In 2017, HBO aired a movie version of the book in which Oprah Winfrey starred in the role of Deborah, Henrietta Lacks' daughter.[6]

This exposure prompted a broad discussion in academic and medical settings of ethical implications related to racial inequities in health care, informed consent, and property rights in human tissue. Lacks and her cells have rarely been explored from a theological perspective. Yet when we studied that story in a classroom mixing divinity school students with those

---

[1] This information comes from the account in Rebecca Skloot, *The Immortal Life of Henrietta Lacks* (New York: Crown Publishers, 2010).
[2] John R. Masters, "Hela Cells 50 Years On: The Good, the Bad and the Ugly," *Nature Reviews. Cancer* 2, no. 4 (2002): 315–19.
[3] "Significant Research Advances Enabled by HeLa Cells," *National Institutes of Health, Office of Science Policy,* https://osp.od.nih.gov/hela-cells/significant-research-advances-enabled-by-hela-cells/.
[4] Ibid.
[5] Norman Foster, "A Cell's Life: The Immortal Life of Henrietta Lacks. (Book Review)," *National Academy of Sciences*, 2010.
[6] George C. Wolfe, "The Immortal Life of Henrietta Lacks," HBO, April 22, 2017.

from medical, nursing, and public health schools, we found that connections and questions poured out in conversation.

Some of these revolved around the striking fact that her cells had attained a kind of immortality. In a genetic and biological sense, she lived on, spread through laboratories around the world. This was a notion in some measure both horrifying and comforting to members of her extended family who only became aware of the survival of her cells years afterward. HeLa cells represented both the promise of industrial laboratory medicine and the poignant significance of one human life whose suffering had become the means to save the lives of many. But the discussion quickly focused even more concretely. The saving benefits that flowed to all of humanity from the painful death of this single obscure person set up echoes of the Christian story. On one hand, it offers a startling exemplification of theological concepts that often remain theoretically abstract. On the other hand, a Christological lens illuminates important dimensions of the Henrietta Lacks' story and its continuing significance.

The ethical aspects of Henrietta Lacks' medical care and its aftermath are of great theological importance. To what extent did she consent for her cells to be shared among scientists? As a Black woman, with a third-grade education, receiving complex cancer care at a bastion of modern medicine, how well did physicians explain her prognosis and her options? Did she receive standard of care?

Family members were completely unaware that Henrietta Lacks' cells were used so widely and to such dramatic effect. No one had informed them. Neither Lacks nor her family received financial recompense for the original specimens or any share in subsequent profits from the innovations developed from her cells. How should her descendants be compensated for the billions of dollars made from the *HeLa* cells? The family only learned of Henrietta Lacks' contributions when scientists reached out to them seeking blood samples to study their DNA. Henrietta Lacks' story raises many issues about patient consent, ownership of one's DNA, the power dynamics between patients and physicians, and racial disparities in our society. Any religion that seeks justice and embodies these principles must engage these questions directly. And they have been the focus of most of the discussion of Lacks' case in recent years.[7]

---

[7] See for instance the lawsuit filed on behalf of Lacks' family. Arseny Shevelev and Georgy Shevelev, "Defending Henrietta Lacks: Justification of Ownership Rights in Separated Human Body Parts," *Vanderbilt Journal of Transnational Law* 55, no. 4 (2022): 957–1005.

The paradoxical features of this story are striking, the contrast between the short disadvantaged life of this poor woman, on the one hand, and the world-changing impact of her cells over the decades that followed. From a strictly genetic Darwinian perspective, Henrietta Lacks is arguably the most successful human being in history. The estimated weight of all the *HeLa* cells exceeds 50 million metric tons.[8] Her DNA has replicated billions of times and is replicating still. Conceived over one hundred years ago, Lacks' unique DNA is approaching the age of the longest-lived human cells and there is no reason to think it will not far surpass that limit. In an age that dreams of immortality in the form of a digital download, she has attained an approximation of it in a tangible and biological shape.

Of course, this is a form of immortality in which the subject herself is deprived of any immediate awareness or participation, while the direct benefits go to numberless others. *HeLa* cells bear her unique DNA, and she lives on after her death in the narrow respect that all of the cells with an individual's DNA normally die with the individual. This "immortality" is not the continuation of person and personality that is presumed in most religious versions of the idea, as well as in those of medical forms of transhumanism that primarily deal with lifespan extension.

The *HeLa* version of immortality is seemingly the exact opposite of attempts at immortality by capturing human consciousness with artificial intelligence and severing it from its biological basis. While her DNA replicates in cellular form, Henrieta Lacks herself is disembodied and lacks consciousness. In her *HeLa* cells, Henrietta has substance but no consciousness. With artificial intelligence, one may have consciousness, but no substance. There is an irony, perhaps a horror, to her immortality. She lives on in cells whose genomic code could, in theory, reconstitute the body she once had. She lives on as a disembodied collection of biochemical reactions, nourished in a petri dish by researchers, at the service to humanity. Her DNA is as enslaved as her ancestors were.

Rebecca Skloot, the author of *The Immortal Life of Henrietta Lacks*, arranged for some extended Lacks family members to meet with a scientist in the lab where he was working with *HeLa* cells.[9] Some of those relatives had believed that Lacks was being held against her will within a medical

---

[8]Fost, "A Cell's Life: The Immortal Life of Henrietta Lacks (Book Review)," 87.
[9]"A Conversation with Rebecca Skloot," WKNO, November 11, 2020, https://www.youtube.com/watch?v=4AuOWSOzdcA&t=1226s.

facility, where scientists performed experiments on her. When the family members held the petri dish in their hands, they spoke to her, as if she might understand. We can identify with their confusion. Henrietta Lacks exists, but in a different form. It is hard for any of us to fully distinguish between biological and personal life or identity.

Questions at the Edge of Medicine and Theology

The mystery of Henrietta Lacks' story is inextricable from the mystery of cancer itself. The cells that live on come from the tumor that killed her. Her cervical cancer was likely caused by an infection of the human papillomavirus (HPV). Decades later, an inoculation against HPV would become part of the standard childhood vaccine series. That vaccine, one of the advances *HeLa* cells supported, may potentially eradicate the very illness that killed her.

She is immortal in this subject-less, biological way through the very diseased mechanism that ended her personal life. It was these cells' unlimited pursuit of their own reproduction that extinguished the larger organism, her body, of which they were a part. Only those of Henrietta Lacks' cells that became cancerous also acquired this extended life that made them vehicles for medical innovation. Her cancer did not simply reveal this unique capacity in those cells; her cancer actually created it. The disease that killed her, led to her peculiar immortality. Whatever good for others may have flowed from that tumor, it was nothing but lethal for Henrietta Lacks and devastating to those that loved her. If she has been an agent of healing to others, it is her own wounding that is the source of the healing.

Cancer is not an invasion from outside: it is a defection in the normal process of a cell's life cycle. Throughout our bodies, cells are constantly dying, releasing their contents in a controlled fashion, and rejuvenating new cells. The scientific word for this is apoptosis, or programmed cell death. It is distinct from necrosis, the death of cells due to injury or external insult. The average adult human loses between 50 and 70 billion cells each day due to apoptosis.[10] The old line from the funeral service in the Book of Common

---

[10] John C. Reed, "Dysregulation of Apoptosis in Cancer," *Journal of Clinical Oncology* 17, no. 9 (1999): 2941–53.

Prayer is very literally true: "in the midst of life we are in death."[11] We live and have health by virtue of strategic dying. In this complex, highly orchestrated process, cells die that others may live. In programmed cell death, cells self-limit in a way that recognizes their interest in the health of the body of which they are a part. Cancer may often partially result from environmental influences, random mutation, or inherited liabilities, but it always expresses itself as a breakdown in the organic polity that makes up the health of our bodies.

Cancer originates in some subset of our own cells that break away from normal biological cooperation. What makes cancer destructive, debilitating, and potentially fatal is the aberration that cells that should die and self-limit do not. Cancer cells seek a kind of self-interest inconsistent with the well-being of the larger body. It is their persistence in replicating without limit that kills the larger organism and so, eventually, the cancer itself. Henrietta Lacks' cancer cells are the exception to this rule, living on long after the body/person of which they had been a part. It is ironic that they do so because they continue to be nourished by a community of researchers, one of whose primary aims is to eliminate cells such as these.

The cancer cells that were preserved from Henrietta Lacks turned out to have nearly miraculous qualities. They did what no other human cells had previously done: reproduce indefinitely in laboratory conditions. These cancer cells had "risen" from the death that is the invariable outcome once they have destroyed their host. The "search" for immortality that functionally drives all cancer was, in this particular case, realized. Indeed, because of this unique quality, one of the ethical questions most debated in relation to Lacks' case is the issue of whether a person ought to have rights and a property interest in cells taken from their body and subsequently used in medical or other kinds of research. Cells removed from human patients in the past had not survived and reproduced long enough to have a utility that raised this question. Cells in organs transplanted from one person to another live on outside their original host. But their benefit is limited to one other body alone, and the process of transplantation has become a highly regulated system with broad institutional oversight.

Even from a purely medical and scientific perspective, Lacks' story pushes us to a frontier where the empirical tends to blend into the philosophical and

---

[11] The Church of England, *The Book of Common Prayer* (New York: Church Publishing Incorporated 2007), 484.

social, raising questions of identity, morality, immortality, and our relation with our own biology. Those who work most directly with cancer, as well as those who suffer from it, often seem led into reflections that go beyond the simply empirical.[12] Modern medical science's long-term struggle with cancer has seen the disappointment of many hopes for definitive solutions. This has led many in that research community to entertain various ways of reimagining the problem, including viewing cancer less on the model of a hostile invader and more on the model of an organism vying for a niche in an environmental ecology. For example, the Cancer Evolution Working Group within the American Association for Cancer Research seeks better prevention and treatment for cancer by understanding its evolution and by viewing cancer as a living organism within the ecology of the human body.[13]

In Lacks' story, the biological mysteries of cancer (a kind of war between our own biological members), the social injustices of racial and economic relations, and the transformative healing power of modern medical technologies all come together in a disorienting mix. This makes us aware of the inadequacy of a simple clinical account of the use of these cells. It calls for a response that integrates all those areas on which it touches so powerfully. Theology is one of those areas. We do not usually think of theology as an experimental science, but the extraordinary story of Henrietta Lacks is an empirical case study that offers an opportunity both to revitalize some theological categories and to benefit from a theological perspective.

Christology and Henrietta Lacks

We have seen the extraordinary questions that swirl around the legacy of Henrietta Lacks and *HeLa* cells. For a Christian, an additional set suggests itself, from the Christological analogies that leap out. Many specific details of her story throw up a profound resonance with Christian language and ideas around Jesus' death. Phrases that appear in medical and journalistic treatments of her story—"rose from the dead," "immortal," "healing for all humanity," "her cells stand in for all human cells"—sound almost more

---

[12]See for instance Siddhartha Mukherjee, *The Emperor of All Maladies: A Biography of Cancer*, 1st Scribner hardcover ed. (New York: Scribner, 2010).
[13]"Cancer Evolution Working Group," American Association for Cancer Research, https://www.aacr.org/professionals/membership/scientific-working-groups/cancer-evolution-working-group/.

theological than scientific, though it is hard empirical data that prompts them. Christians believe that the death of Jesus Christ has a saving effect for all of us. Those who unite in faith with Jesus will receive new life, even eternal life, and reconciliation with God and neighbor. Those with faith in modern medicine, who receive *HeLa* derivatives into themselves, in the form of vaccines or therapeutics, have a promise of extended life and reduced morbidity. Through Henrietta Lacks' disease and death, laboratory science has used her cells to save the lives of millions.

We can speak of Christological analogies in two broad perspectives. In one, the extraordinary features of Henrietta Lacks' story offer interpretive and communicative metaphors that deepen the expression of traditional Christian teachings, particularly in terms of the web of relations through which the incarnation works. Her story undergirds our understanding of Christ. In the other perspective, it is the story of Christ that illuminates our approach to Henrietta Lacks, calling out aspects of this story that are lost in a purely medical or instrumental understanding, because the comparison with Christ focuses our attention on the individual at the center.

In expressing the saving power they found in Christ's death and resurrection, early Christians turned to a variety of metaphors: ransom out of slavery, healing of sickness, defeat of the power of death, escape from the devil and forces of evil. One of the early church writers, Athanasius, summed up his sense of the incarnation as healing human nature. By taking on a body like ours, God would turn humans "again toward incorruption, and quicken them from death by the assumption of his body and by the grace of the resurrection, banishing death from them like straw from the fire."[14]

In these images, Christians were grasping for ways to express a fundamental conviction: God's incarnation in Jesus, including his death and resurrection, was of universal, saving human significance. All of the images reached to express this: a single ransom is paid to release all the slaves; a victory is won over the power that holds all captive. Threaded through many of these images was repeated reference to blood. This was understandable, both because there was long familiarity with the use of blood in religious rituals of commitment and expiation, as for instance in animal sacrifices, and because human blood evoked a profound sense of awe, since it was clearly essential to life and its appearance in any quantity was associated with great peril as well as with fertility and blessing, menstruation, and childbirth.

---

[14] St. Athanasius, *On the Incarnation of the Word* (London: David Nutt, 1885), 13.

Clearly organic and biological, ideas about blood funded what we might call the primary *medical* interpretation of Christian redemption. It was the fact that all humans shared the same created nature and shared the same blood that helped make intelligible the idea of a universal saving act in one on behalf of all. If God's presence in Jesus was to change all people, Jesus' humanity had to be in full solidarity with all humanity. Ideas about the power of blood bridged both mystical and medical categories. They were used in reference to the effect of Jesus' death. In Heb. 12:24, Jesus is spoken of as mediator of a new covenant, through "sprinkled blood that speaks a better word than the blood of Abel." Blood had long been used to seal human covenants and contracts. The blood of Abel, who had been murdered by his brother, "cried out from the ground" for justice or vengeance. The blood called for the covenant of retribution to be carried out. By contrast, the blood of Jesus was seen as the seal on a covenant whose terms demanded mercy and not revenge. These references demonstrate the importance of blood in signifying a universal human unity.

If early Christians had understood human biology more extensively, they might have found the blood image even more apt. If they had known that there is such a thing as a universal donor—one particular type of blood, found in some but not in all, that can be universally received by all to healing or "saving" effect—they would have been delighted. In their view, the incarnation was just that kind of saving particularity, a transfusion into the common blood bank of humankind carrying healing antibodies. Athanasius wrote, explaining why the human condition could not be changed by fiat from outside, "If death was within the body, woven into its very substance and dominating it as though completely one with it, the need was for Life to be woven into it instead, so that the body, by enduing itself with life, might cast corruption off."[15]

Redemption is carried on from the inside out, and its realization in humans—individually and collectively—works the same way. Athanasius regards the incarnation as an ontological change in the condition of all humanity. But that changed possibility has to be appropriated or adopted by people through faith and commitment to become fully effective in their lives. By deeper participation in unity with Christ, more and more of the divine life and will in Christ becomes part of us, or actually renews what we

---

[15]Athanasius, *On the Incarnation: The Treatise De Incarnatione Verbi Dei* (Crestwood, NY: St. Vladimir's Seminary Press, 1998), 80–1.

already are, restoring the health that is rooted in creation. The eucharist or communion is a sacramental form of this transfusion, just as actions of love and justice "in the way of Jesus" are other forms of transfusion.

We can see then how these ancient convictions, often bound up in images that are not intuitive or immediate for us, resonate with the facts of Henrietta Lacks' story. We could even see aspects of the Eucharist in *HeLa* cells. A vaccine that we receive contains elements or proteins from *HeLa* cells, and so we take into ourselves a small piece of Henrietta Lacks. The parallels are haunting. It is not her blood but her tissue, her cervical cells that are the source of healing. The DNA of those cells is unique to her person, and to her womanhood. Yet it is their identity with all human cells that make them the source of cures and treatments that function for us all.

Henrietta Lacks lives today, her life spread increasingly across the world, and its effects have literally become a healing part of our bodies. It is because Henrietta Lacks' cells are human that they can be the source of cures that work for all. Only one who shares our nature can be saving for us in this way. It is that combination of shared identity with us and a quality unique to her—the continuous life of her cells—that makes her legacy saving. *HeLa* cells created a new condition in human life, one that now applies to all humanity. But it requires active response to that possibility on the part of researchers with the tools of modern medicine, and then individual decisions, for people to participate in the healing benefits—by accepting vaccination, for instance. We can say that by her affliction, we have all been healed.

One of the marginal and despised, who died unremarked, rejected, and under conditions of oppression, she has become a "chief cornerstone" of our medical world.[16] From death, she was raised in a literal bodily resurrection, though not a personal one. She does not just live on in the memories of her loved ones, but as an active presence in the world with tangible effects.

In all these ways, Rebecca Lacks' story illuminates the Christian one. In prior ages, Christians reached for analogies that could explain that their experience of Jesus' impact, while extraordinary in nature, had parallels in the world we knew. Henrietta Lacks and her cells are such an analogy. Christ is like Henrietta Lacks, in the sense that she links an individual death with new life, a unique identity with benefit to all humanity, as Christians believe

---

[16]Psalm 118:22–23, quoted in Matthew 21:42. "The stone that the builders rejected has become the chief cornerstone. This is marvelous in our eyes."

Christ also does. Just as the early church found powerful imagery based on the understanding of blood in that time, so we may find the terms of this extraordinary medical saga offering very modern imagery for Christ's redemptive work.

These resonances demonstrate that the medical realm may offer us images of theological power. But they are not lifted up to erase Henrietta Lacks from her own story, as though she is nothing but an illustration. To focus on Henrietta Lacks simply as a heuristic image to articulate Christian beliefs about Jesus would be a response in the theological realm no different from the way the medical world seized upon her cells' usefulness while ignoring her story and forgetting her name.

If Christ is like Henrietta Lacks, and the comparison is a way of expressing Christian experience or belief, it is also true that Henrietta Lacks is like Christ, with the comparison also being a way of expressing her value in her own right, and recognizing the challenge her story poses. In this sense, Christ is the illustration, and she is the one to be highlighted. The manner of Jesus' death and suffering has a perennial power to raise up and empower people in victimized situations.

That is to say, God's presence in the rejected and marginalized Jesus has the capacity to sensitize us also to anyone who is placed in a similar condition. In this sense, we are to look not so much at Jesus, as at the one the awareness of his story allows us to see, and calls us to respect. The analogy lifts up her particular personhood. Recalling her importance, honoring and respecting her presence in this larger narrative of medical healing, is another kind of rescue and resurrection, one that resonates with the vindication of the crucified one. In this way too, their stories fit together.[17]

Just as Christ's resurrection made it impossible to ignore the way he died, when without it he would have been erased as his executioners intended, so the fact of the continuing life and effect of Lacks' cells *should* make it impossible to forget her actual life: who she was and what happened to her. But clearly that recognition did not come readily and required a spiritual or moral sensitivity. In addition to the medical healing that Lacks enabled, we could say she has also become the source of a moral and social regeneration when we attend to the implications of her treatment as an African American

---

[17]For more on this function of the cross, see S. Mark Heim, "Their Cross Problem and Ours: Thoughts on the Aesthetic of Crucifixion," *Interpretation* 76, no. 1 (2022): 27–38.

woman, the lessons to be learned for medical practice, and for medical policy about ownership and control over bodily tissues.

Comparisons with Christ could function as a kind of romantic obscuration, whose only interest is in the healing effects that flowed from her suffering. To the contrary, one thing the analogy should do is suggest that just as the transformative effect of Jesus' resurrection requires a reckoning with the forces that brought about his rejection and death, so recognition of the healing benefits that flow from Henrietta Lacks' life requires us to look back at the facts of that life, of the racism and oppression of that time, of the powers of sin and death to which she was subject, and from which our society as well as our bodies need healing. Christ's death, whatever good flows from it, was due to the oppression of an occupying government, to the betrayal or abandonment by trusted companions, and to human sin. And a major good that does flow from the cross is precisely recognition of such social evils and our participation in them, and action to overcome these. Henrietta Lacks' death was set in a context of oppression, one that denied her access to health care on the same basis as others and denied her recognition after death.

In drawing the comparison, we underline the sense in which her story belongs to a wider history of African Americans abused or mis-served by the medical system in the United States, such as those in the Tuskegee syphilis study.[18] In fact, the specific medical discipline charged with caring for Henrietta Lacks, gynecology, was pioneered in the United States by doctors who performed operations without anesthesia (a technology then available) on enslaved women.[19] Her story comes out of a narrative of oppression and systemic racism. To see her as a source of healing, similar to Jesus, is also to raise the question of what it is we need healing from, a question that points us directly at the elements of our society in need of transformation.

The tensions implicit in making such a comparison reflect tensions present in theology itself. Recent theological discussions of Jesus' death have been deeply shaped by Delores Williams and her womanist critique of surrogacy.[20] She states that theology that makes of Jesus' death an ideal for

---

[18] William J. Curran, "The Tuskegee Syphilis Study," *The New England Journal of medicine* 289, no. 14 (1973): 730–1.
[19] Deirdre Cooper Owens, *Medical Bondage: Race, Gender, and the Origins of American Gynecology* (Athens, GA: University of Georgia Press, 2017).
[20] Delores S. Williams, *Sisters in the Wilderness: The Challenge of Womanist God-Talk* (Maryknoll, NY: Orbis Books, 1993).

others to emulate, by embracing suffering and bearing the sins of others, reinforces an existing cultural assumption that already has made such "service" an obligatory role for Black women. This is particularly so in regard to the surrogacy in which Black women were economically compelled to care for the children (as nannies), the households (as cooks and maids), or the sick (as nurses and health aides) of others, while they were unable to adequately do the same for their own families. The way that Lacks' cells have been put ceaselessly to work in laboratories around the world as stand-ins for all human cells, without recognition or recompense, is an uncomfortable mirror of other forms of coerced surrogacy. From Williams' perspective, it is Jesus' teaching about justice and equality that should be heart of Christian belief rather than any redemptive value in his death.

James Cone, a pioneer of Black liberation theology, acknowledged the importance of this insight but argued that it left aside the profound meaning the cross held for the dispossessed and oppressed.[21] In it, they saw an accurate representation of their suffering condition, and an affirmation that God was on the side of the victim, identifying with their struggle. In celebrating Christ's defeat of death, Christians do not endorse what killed him, but testify to his innocence. In appreciating the good that has flowed from Henrietta Lacks' cancer, we must simultaneously recognize that she was denied the agency to choose her path and also denied the opportunity to participate in the good that her affliction made possible.

In this sense, she is a kind of antitype of Jesus, and joining their stories also invites us to see these differences. Living on in the replication of her cells is only an ersatz version of what Christians mean by resurrection, precisely because it excludes her from that redemption as a conscious, personal participant. This is something the Christian hope cherishes for her still. Indeed, resurrection, and not immortality, is the nature of Christian hope. Immortality has to do with self-sufficiency, an immunity to death, that separates what is permanent and enduring from what is regarded as material and transient. Resurrection is not a denial of or escape from death, but a new reality on the other side of it, one dependent on relation and on a renewal of material creation. Immortality is about preservation. But resurrection is about transformation, and to some extent about restitution.

Lacks was not intentionally put to death and had no anticipation of what might flow from that death. In her life and dying, she lacked the agency

---

[21]James H. Cone, *The Cross and the Lynching Tree* (Maryknoll, NY: Orbis Books, 2011).

available to Jesus. Nor did she have to give her life to have a redemptive effect on humanity. Samples were taken from her cervical tumor in the process of treatment, and those cells were already proliferating in their extraordinary manner in George Gey's laboratory, and being passed on to other labs, by the time Lacks died. If her cancer had been cured and her life saved, she could have lived on both in person and in biological research. Of course, the very qualities that made her cells uniquely valuable in research were the same that made them extremely difficult to eliminate from her body.

In Memory of Her

The gospel account of Jesus has strong notes of reversal and vindication. The one who is lowly and rejected becomes an honored foundation. Henrietta Lacks' story has this note as well. A person so humble and unremarked during her life is understood to have become crucially important. In the face of her social marginalization and her early death from an aggressive disease, the cells that bear the mark of her personal identity stubbornly persist. They support ever-renewed forms of healing and save the lives of millions of people.

It is a narrative of triumph out of tragedy, but also of imponderable circumstances. Of all the places Henrietta Lacks could have gone for care, she presented to one of the only medical research hospitals in the country, one with research facilities down the hall. Had she arrived virtually anywhere else, her cells would have been used for diagnosis only, then discarded as medical waste, their exceptional qualities never known and their benefits never realized. The use of *HeLa* cells is a triumph of human ingenuity and modern medicine. But that use is also enmeshed in the murkier ethical world of profit-driven pharmaceutical companies, powerful academic institutions, and endemic racial injustice. In her single life, these vast principalities and powers, creative skills, and fallen structures all intersect.

After the fact, recognition and acknowledgment of her have begun to catch up with the substantive effect of her legacy. To commemorate her life, Johns Hopkins University convenes an academic lecture series in her honor.[22]

---

[22]"The Henrietta Lacks Memorial Lecture Series," *Johns Hopkins Institute for Clinical & Translational Research*, https://ictr.johnshopkins.edu/community-engagement/programs/henrietta-lacks-memorial-lecture/.

Members of her family now sit on a board of advisors to direct the research in which *HeLa* cells will be used.[23] These gestures, books and movies, and the growing attention to her story across many disciplines reinscribe her role in the scientific saga from which she had been erased. With that recognition comes renewed appreciation for dimensions of justice, gratitude, and human suffering that should always be part of the scientific medical enterprise, but are too often missing.

In October of 2024, Johns Hopkins University and Medical School broke ground on the Henrietta Lacks building, which will house both academic medical research and the study of the ethics governing that research itself. The university president said that the building was a "concrete commitment to ensure that Henrietta Lacks' name will be as immortal as her cells."[24]

Rebecca Skloot wrote that only one person she interviewed from the Johns Hopkins hospital staff, who served there at the time, remembered whether George Gey (the research scientist who cultured her cells) and Henrietta Lacks ever actually met or spoke. One of Gey's colleagues recalled Gey saying he had visited her after seeing the extraordinary replication of her cells. He told her that her cells would make her immortal and help save the lives of countless people. She smiled and "told him she was glad her pain would come to some good for someone."[25] We can hope the small window of recognition and participation, carried by that fragile memory, was some foretaste of what the resurrected life might yet hold for her.

That hope is a religious one. But it has a practical correlative. The Gospel of Mark includes the story of an unnamed woman who pours out a costly salve to anoint Jesus. He responds with a promise: "wherever this gospel is preached throughout the world, what she has done will also be told, in memory of her."[26] It is a small sign of healing that so long as the medical effects of Henrietta Lacks' life continue to spread, from generation to generation, the story of their origin in her life may continue to be told, in memory of her.

---

[23]"NIH, Lacks Family Reach Understanding to Share Genomic Data of HeLa Cells," *National Institutes of Health*, August 7, 2013, https://www.nih.gov/news-events/news-releases/nih-lacks-family-reach-understanding-share-genomic-data-hela-cells.
[24]See https://www.hopkinsmedicine.org/news/newsroom/news-releases/2024/10/johns-hopkins-and-family-of-henrietta-lacks-break-ground-on-building-named-in-honor-of-henrietta-lacks.
[25]Skloot, *The Immortal Life of Henrietta Lacks*, 66.
[26]Mark 14:9, New International Version.

References

Athanasius. *On the Incarnation: The Treatise De Incarnatione Verbi Dei*. Crestwood, NY: St. Vladimirs Seminary Press, 1998.

Athanasius, St. *On the Incarnation of the Word*. London: David Nutt, 1885.

Cone, James H. *The Cross and the Lynching Tree*. Maryknoll, NY: Orbis Books, 2011.

Cooper Owens, Deirdre. *Medical Bondage: Race, Gender, and the Origins of American Gynecology*. Athens, GA: University of Georgia Press, 2017.

Curran, William J. "The Tuskegee Syphilis Study." [In English]. *The New England Journal of Medicine* 289, no. 14 (1973): 730–1.

England, The Church of. *The Book of Common Prayer*. New York: Church Publishing Incorporated, 2007.

Fost, Norman. "A Cells Life: The Immortal Life of Henrietta Lacks (Book Review)." 87: *National Academy of Sciences*, 2010.

Heim, S. Mark. "Their Cross Problem and Ours: Thoughts on the Aesthetic of Crucifixion." *Interpretation* 76, no. 1 (2022): 27–38.

Masters, John R. "Hela Cells 50 Years On: The Good, the Bad and the Ugly." [In English]. *Nature Reviews. Cancer* 2, no. 4 (2002): 315–19.

Mukherjee, Siddhartha. *The Emperor of All Maladies: A Biography of Cancer*. 1st Scribner hardcover ed. New York: Scribner, 2010.

Reed, John C. "Dysregulation of Apoptosis in Cancer." [In English]. *Journal of Clinical Oncology* 17, no. 9 (1999): 2941–53.

Shevelev, Arseny, and Georgy Shevelev. "Defending Henrietta Lacks: Justification of Ownership Rights in Separated Human Body Parts." [In English]. *Vanderbilt Journal of Transnational Law* 55, no. 4 (2022): 957–1005.

Skloot, Rebecca. *The Immortal Life of Henrietta Lacks*. New York: Crown Publishers, 2010.

Williams, Delores S. *Sisters in the Wilderness: The Challenge of Womanist God-Talk*. Maryknoll, NY: Orbis Books, 1993.

Wolfe, George C. "The Immortal Life of Henrietta Lacks." HBO, April 22, 2017.

Epilogue

Last Things and First Things

When Ben interviews applicants for his residency program, he asks a single question, "What is the One Thing?" He gives them the question the evening before so that they can think about it. Which requires a brief explanation. "The One Thing" comes from the movie, *City Slickers*. Billy Crystal plays a middle-aged dad who is in a suburban existential crises. With some friends, he leaves his placid life, and goes on a cattle drive out West.

He meets an old leathery cowboy, played perfectly by Jack Palance, who says, "I've met you guys before. You think this cattle drive will save your life. It won't. The secret to life is the One Thing."

Billy Crystal asks, "Tell me, what is the one thing?"

Palance responds, "That is for you to figure out for yourself."

Soon after, the cowboy dies, and Crystal and the other tenderfoot ranch hands are left to bring the cattle safely home. They strive. They conquer. Happy ending.

Ben asks the question because he is searching for the inner architecture of the physician-to-be. He reports, "This has been a deeply moving experience each year. I interview extremely talented, accomplished people, on their best behavior. I'm also on my best behavior. I am privileged to hear powerful testimonies about the most important aspect of people's lives. I have heard hundreds of "one things." I have heard about important values—faith, family, community, love, connection, curiosity. I have heard about deeply moving experiences—the death of family members, the surprise of love, the jolt of intellectual curiosity."

At this point, to project how someone will function as a doctor, it is no longer helpful to explore the nuts and bolts of medicine. It is more helpful to explore how medicine itself fits into the "one big thing" in their lives, the larger vision.

How the Healing Happens

Ben's favorite response comes not from an applicant, but from the second-century church writer Irenaeus, who said "The glory of God is a human being fully alive."[1] Medicine, at its best, allows us to live, with the fullest use of our physical capacities. Spirituality and theology give us a vision of what the outer boundary of flourishing might be, how to live and what to live for. Together, theology and medicine share that hope to flourish as human beings, to be fully alive. In doing so, in living fully, we give glory to God.

The answer to Ben's question is important in making good doctors, as it is in making good priests or pastors. We believe the medical vocation is most fully healing when it makes space for the one big thing in those it treats. Whether in regard to end-of-life care, or control of chronic pain, or overcoming addiction, there is no sound plan of treatment that does not include among its vital signs the patient's own measure of what health and flourishing mean to them.

One of our colleagues headed up a neighborhood clinic, serving those in a poverty-ridden area of the city. She noticed that for a large majority of the people they treated, religion and spirituality, of various sorts, played a large role in their lives and in their response to illness. For their medical records, patients were questioned extensively about what medications they took regularly, including substances like heroin or marijuana, but extending to every vitamin and herbal supplement, the quantities of coffee and tea. It was ironic to her that there was not even a cursory interest in what these people's daily spiritual or religious diet might be. She set out to include such information as part of a patient history, if for no other purpose than to communicate that this part of their lives was seen rather than ignored. That alone, she believed, would improve residents' utilization of the clinic and the effectiveness of their treatment there.

We have enough experience to know that religion-as-medicine, at least as a replacement for or competitor with allopathic medicine, is a bad idea in terms of physical health outcomes. Religion included as a dimension within medicine, as we have described, is a good idea in medical terms. Our experience with medicine-as-religion, treating the body as machinery and taking its ideal health and beauty to be the content of our salvation, is of

---

[1]Irenaeus *Against Heresies*, IV, 35, 7.

shorter duration. It has given us much for which to be grateful, turning many cancers and HIV from death sentences into chronic diseases.

The problem with medicine-as-religion is that it fails at the exact moment when we need it most. When ideal physical outcomes are not possible, medicine lacks the vocabulary and often lacks the emotional architecture, to offer true holistic care. There is no pathway to love in medicine, only another therapeutic intervention. This why theology is so critical for the practice of medicine. Theology gives the language, the intellectual and spiritual structure to embrace our full humanity. Forgiveness, reconciliation, and purpose are precisely what robust theology offers.

One question comes back to us again and again in our conversations. How does the healing happen? Sometimes, healing happens when the heart valve is replaced, the skin cancer excised, or the appendix removed. In such cases, we might even be able to say with some confidence how the biological healing works, down to a molecular level. Sometimes, healing happens when a community joins forces to overcome a pandemic. Sometimes, healing happens when a mystical certainty or an overpowering love flow into a person whose medical condition is never going to improve. Sometimes healing happens when friends lower their buddy through the roof to get to someone who might be able to help, and Jesus says, "Get up. Take your mat and go home."[2] To limit healing to a bodily function or a spiritual condition, distorts both medicine and theology.

Medical care, like spiritual care, is at its best when the "one big thing" of the caregiver meets the "one big thing" of the patient. By which we don't intend to say they should share the same religious beliefs or practices, or even address those with great specificity. We picture instead that the significance that medicine has for the doctor practicing it intersects with the meaning of the well-being sought by their patient. A doctor may be devoted to the self-determination of her patients, for instance, not as an institutional imposition, but as a deep human value. This is part of what makes medicine more than a job for her. Her patient may be someone of deep Jewish or Buddhist commitment. The nature of the doctor's spirituality and that of her patient are not the same, but they can reinforce each other because they meet on a terrain that is itself more than a strictly medical one. Much of the time, that intersection may be a routine and hardly noticeable feature, hardly the subject of deep or explicit conversation. Recovery from today's pneumonia

---

[2]Luke 5:24.

may fit easily, and without much need for reflection, into the vision both doctor and patient have of human flourishing. Faith and visions of human flourishing come to the fore particularly in times of crisis. But, as we have described, they are clearly in play even in rather prosaic medical interactions such as taking a medication or following a doctor's instructions.

Brave New World

Our concern in this book has been how religion and medicine may fit together in the texture of medicine as it is. What is the big picture for the health effects of religious observance? How may spiritual resources figure concretely in supporting health and recovery? We think all the topics we have discussed will have continuing relevance for a long time. But we are also aware that "normal" is shifting ground, and nowhere more so than in health care.

Until very recently, medicine has been confined to "fixing what is broken." We have occasionally pointed out that medicine has begun to move into another realm, into granting human beings capacities that they have never had before. Immunities gained through vaccination, or resistance to infections granted by antibiotics, could plausibly be said to be new human conditions, transformations of our natures. But these seem more continuous with our existing characteristics than other changes now on the horizon. Medicine is on the edge of an era in which it will not only heal our infirmities, but perhaps create new forms of humanity.

Electronic stimulators and neural network links have been surgically implanted into patients who are paralyzed, with some positive effects. Tools to vocalize have been used for years by people who have lost their ability to speak. Treatments like these, extraordinary as they are, seek to "level up" to standards of health that are common for most people. But there is no neat line that distinguishes the replacement knee, "as good as new," from a bionic or genetic enhancement with capacities no one is born with or can achieve naturally. Similarly, drugs developed to mitigate cognitive or physical deficits can be deployed for enhancement and transcendence of what is "normal."

In this connection, the theology-medicine conversation becomes more explicit, as the practice of medicine leads us into areas that necessarily raise philosophical and moral questions. The Program for Medicine, Spirituality, and Religion at Yale convenes a group of graduate students several times a year to consider salient questions at the intersection of medicine and religion. It is not a bad rule of thumb that if you want to know about the future of a field, you should listen more to the interests of students and graduate students than those of senior faculty. By that measure, this conversation is headed into deeper waters.

Our group gathers at a renowned pizza establishment near campus (In New Haven, debates about which pizza joint is best are often more heated than those over religion, politics, or anything else). We toss around ideas, share research projects, and consider friction points between the worlds of medicine and religion. In recent months the great debates have revolved around personhood. Could a chatbot or an AI program be a person? This led into discussion of souls and "ensoulment" in religious views, of debates over whether organic bodies are essential attributes of persons. Can minds, spirits, souls be transplanted?

One in the group came up with a hypothetical scenario. Many children each year are born anencephalic, without a cerebral cortex and with only a functioning brainstem. The child respires, takes nourishment, circulates blood through the body, but for all practical purposes has no higher cortical function. Despite this, most consider that child a person, one with an inherent dignity. We cannot imagine a priest or pastor who would not baptize the infant.

What if an artificially intelligent chatbot could be transplanted into this entity? Already, we have limited brain transplants of different sorts. Is not an artificial cerebral cortex merely an extension of such devices? This chatbot would receive inputs of sight, sense, and smell from the child's brainstem functions and generate ideas about these inputs. The chatbot would have a personality, of sorts. We could interact with this person, befriend this person. Is this a redemption of the child, of the sort that religious faith might imagine happening in some future heavenly realm?

Another debate about persons came not from the computer side but the biological one. It will soon be possible to string genes together to make a forty-six chromosome nucleus and place that package into an undifferentiated stem cell, which, in theory, could be placed into an artificial womb. Gene splicing and stem cell technologies already exist and are evolving rapidly. Artificial womb technology is under development and shows promise to care for infants born very prematurely. Theoretically, a human stem cell could be placed into a pig or chimpanzee uterus. If such a forty-six chromosome entity were born, who would its parents be? There would be no donor egg or sperm. The constructed stem cell would have been knit together from extant fragments of DNA. The womb could be artificial.

The debates in this group are intense because although these are presently research topics, they may ultimately become medical questions, and then procedures to be carried out by caregivers. Doctors will be expected to administer treatments that are transformations. These will stretch our understanding of what counts as a patient and what counts as a treatment.

Ethical considerations are important here. The four pillars of biomedical ethics—benevolence, non-malfeasance, justice, and autonomy—are critical to evaluate how technology impacts personhood.[3] But before ethical considerations can even be applied, theological and philosophical questions of personhood must be resolved. If a constructed forty-six chromosome entity is not a person, we can ask whether it is ethical to harvest its organs for transplantation. But if it deserves the dignity of personhood, the ethical norms that apply are those for patients.

Many of today's most controversial areas of medicine appear on this emerging boundary between therapy and enhancement, cure and transformation. An example would be the arguments over gender affirming care for trans-identified young people, which have recently become prominent among medical associations in the United States and Europe.[4] The range of treatments in question can be understood from one perspective as "mere treatment," in the framework of therapeutic responses to the pain and struggles of persons who experience incongruity between their bodies and their self-understanding. Treatments, from psychological therapy through a range of medications and surgeries, are in this sense an attempt to return someone to a base line level of well-being. Those same interventions can also be seen as a kind of transformation, a perspective that underlines the novelty of the end state, the permanent alignment of physiology with gender identity in adolescents. To combine medications and techniques (puberty blocking drugs, cross sex hormones, and gender reassignment surgeries) in a manner that only recently became medically feasible, is to create something that strictly speaking has not existed before. It is a sort of

---

[3] Tom L. Beauchamp and James F. Childress, *Principles of Biomedical Ethics*, 8th ed. (New York: Oxford University Press, 2019).

[4] For instance, see the recent positive and negative responses to the Cass Report, produced for the National Health Service in the United Kingdom by pediatrician Hilary Cass. The report itself can be found here Hilary Cass, "The Cass Review: Independent Review of Gender Identity Services for Children and Young People," *National Health Service, UK*, https://cass.independent-review.uk/home/publications/final-report/.

new creation. Some view it as a liberating and healing creation, just as we might say that life-long insulin dependent healthy diabetics are something that never existed before medical discoveries. Some view it as more experimental and problematic, even abusive, in running the risk of damaging natural capacities for fertility and sexual function. One can see this as "normal medicine" and either oppose it as mistaken treatment or support it as valid treatment. One can see it as a new creation, and endorse it or condemn it. Our point is that more and more medical questions are moving into the latter category.

The pizza debates always include a strong dose of popular culture references. In 1984, the movie *The Terminator* told the incredible story of a cyborg who travels back in time to murder a pregnant woman, Sarah Connor. Her son will grow up to become the leader of the human resistance against Skynet, the omniscient, all-powerful computer network which gained self-awareness in the future and took over the world, exterminating most humans. Skynet has sent a cyborg back in time to prevent John Connor's birth and therefore the annoying human rebellion.

Students were not only interested in the premise—can a computer be conscious?—but also liked to play with the question: what developments that are now underway might future versions of ourselves want to come back in time to prevent?

New Last Things

One branch of Christian theology we have not mentioned much in this book is eschatology, the doctrine of the "last things."[5] This considers the final destiny not only of individual persons, in life beyond death, but of all history and creation: the "new heaven and new earth" where God's aims are fulfilled. It would appear far removed from our theology and medicine discussion, save perhaps in connection with the topic of death and dying. But just as the human capacity to generate global "end of the world" scenarios through nuclear war or the devastation of nature increasingly evokes eschatological

---

[5] A good basic text is Jürgen Moltmann and Margaret Kohl, The Coming of God: Christian Eschatology (Minneapolis, MN: Fortress Press,, 2004), https://yale.idm.oclc.org/login?URL=http:/
/www.aspresolver.com/aspresolver.asp?TCR1;1868645.

language in our political and scientific discourse, so the scope of modern medicine suggests its relevance as well.

For most of human history, eschatological, religious thinking drove the outer boundaries of imagination about human flourishing, even in the biological sense. No more sickness, no more pain, no more war: there was no conceivable, practical path to such outcomes. The visions arose nonetheless, images of human flourishing that offered a transcendent standard of judgment. In many ways, medical research and technology have moved into a similar space. This stretches our sense of possibility, and it may also make our eschatological visions of human good more relevant and practical. Such religious modes of thinking may play an important role in helping us come to terms with new medical realities, individually and culturally.

The doctrine has always been subject to disagreement over the mode in which this radical future comes to us: by incremental, historical progress, or by catastrophic upheaval, or on an unseen spiritual plane. Eschatology has both a negative and a positive side. On the negative side are judgment and apocalypse, the dramatic and sometimes violent clearing away of what stands in the way of human fulfilment. On the positive side are renewal and transformation into the kingdom of God. The work of salvation is the work of healing what is broken, but also of building or growing what has never yet been. It has an "already and not yet" character. The "not yet" refers to the ultimate horizon of the end of history as we know it. The "already" refers to signs, the "inbreaking" or first fruits of that final possibility that begin to be discerned here and now. The incarnation of Christ is the central example of such anticipatory inbreaking, a coincidence of the end times and present history, but signs include events of social and individual transformation as well.

Christian thinking about this hope includes the flourishing of our bodily natures. "The lame walk and the blind see" is reported as one infallible sign of the kingdom's presence, as too that the poor are fed and the oppressed freed. In this respect, the work of healing is not just an act of neighborly care or of compassion. It is a sign of divine presence, the manifestation of history's true direction. As we have seen (for instance with Hildegard's medieval medicine), medical care has in this way always fit as a Christian practice, an aspect of the "already" dimension of salvation.

This is an important point in relation to medical eschatology. The Christian final things place justice, community, and communion on the same footing as bodily well-being as marks of human flourishing. The hesitation about medical technology has to do with whether it leads to flourishing in those respects. The latest biomedical breakthrough is most often the prize for the rich and connected. The poor and disenfranchised are often the ones digging in the mines for the precious metals for our medical technology, or serving as the test subjects in the randomized controlled trials that more and more often take place in poorer countries. Technology can enhance the human flourishing of a few but can leave many behind.

For Christians, it is a matter of discernment. *The Terminator* makes new technology a doomsday scenario. Our instincts are to exercise caution as new technology becomes available. But there is much about which we can be hopeful. These new technologies are products of intellect, curiosity, and a passion to cure, which are themselves gifts from God, however many other more sordid motives may be intermingled. Being creators is part of what it means to be in the divine image. The challenge is how to incorporate new technology into our human flourishing. It is to ask, "Does this new creation enhance human dignity and community?" Or even, "How do we glorify God in these creations?"

What should be regarded as redemptive transformation, part of the eschatological fulfillment of humanity, even if it goes where no historical human has ever gone before? And what should be seen as likely to draw us in a dystopian and even apocalyptic direction? Even within the realm of healing, fixing what is broken, there are limitations: physical restorations that come at too high a moral or spiritual cost, causes and purposes whose value is such as to make health itself a secondary good. In the uncharted territory of transhumanism these concerns dramatically multiply.

For believers in eschatological change, it can never be a decisive objection that some new possibility transcends humanity as we have known it. Such is exactly the nature of their hope. The question is what counts as fulfillment or realization and what may be a denial or a distortion of our existing humanity and of the ultimate hope. At our meeting, the pizza is finished. The conversation is not. Our group disperses. Residents and chaplains will go back to their work in the hospital, divinity students back to the bedsides and sanctuaries and social service organizations of their weekly rounds. As students and teachers, we all return to the shared work of reading and writing and thinking. To which many of us add prayer, meditation, or worship. These conversations themselves are part of what keeps medicine humane and religion relevant.

Looking toward the future is stimulating, sobering, and humbling. But today's tasks are enough for today. We hope readers adopt nurturing the healthy partnership of religion and medicine as one of those tasks. Insofar as we do that, we believe we will be better prepared for the challenges to come.

References

Beauchamp, Tom L., and James F. Childress. *Principles of Biomedical Ethics*. Eighth ed. New York: Oxford University Press, 2019.

Cass, Hilary. "The Cass Review: Independent Review of Gender Identity Services for Children and Young People." *National Health Service, UK*. https://cass.independent-review.uk/home/publications/final-report/.

Moltmann, Jürgen, and Margaret Kohl. *The Coming of God Christian Eschatology*. Minneapolis, MN: Fortress Press, 2004. https://yale.idm.oclc.org/login?URL=http://www.aspresolver.com/aspresolver.asp?TCR1;1868645.

Index

Note: Page numbers followed by 'n' indicate note number(s).

acceptance
   and anxiety 162–4
   conscious 103
   social 42
addiction 167–81
   forgiveness as a health issue 178–81
   medical models 174–8
   treatment that looks like a church 170–4
AIDS 154–7
Alcoholics Anonymous (AA) 170–2
"alert" function of pain 84
alternative medicine 75
American Association for Cancer Research 209
American Psychological Association 185
Ancient Greek philosophy 196
Angels in America 157–60
anti-inflammatory processes 77
anxiety and acceptance 162–4
apophatic way of approaching God 10
Aquinas, Thomas 115
Aristotle 46, 196
art of dying 96–102
Aurelius, Marcus 196

bad death 99
Battle of Borodino 134
Beauvoir, Simone de 162
Beckett, Samuel 190
   Waiting for Godot 190
bedside prayer tool 81
Being Mortal (Gawande) 95
black bile 48–9

Black liberation theology 215
Blue Zones of Happiness: Lessons from the World's Happiest People, The (Buettner) 124
Britton, Willoughby 112
Buber, Martin 163
   I and Thou 163
Buddhism 5 n.5, 112, 125
Buettner, Daniel 124
   Blue Zones of Happiness: Lessons from the World's Happiest People, The 124
burnout
   flourishing 192–5
   in physicians and clergy 184–8
   responses to 188–9
   as spiritual crisis 183–98
   way forward 195–8
Burnt Out Case, The (Greene) 183, 186

calling 30–2
   face of 30–2
   and obligation 26–30
Camus, Albert
   Plague, The 140
cancer 207–8
   and Christology 203–17
   and immortality 203–17
Cancer Evolution Working Group 209
care 35–7
caregiver 83, 221. *See also* religious patient
Carnegie Foundation 55
cataphatic way of approaching God 10
Catholic Church 183

"Celebrate Recovery" 172
cholesterol-lowering medications 107
Christian 137–8, 143
  belief 85–6, 98
  beliefs and practices 137
  confessional traditions 115
  culture 93
  devotion 136
  encouragement of self-
    examination 99
  faith 97
  hope 215
  ideal of art 103
  medicine 51
  practice 83
  redemption 211
  social networks 138
  spirituality 93
  theology 10, 86, 115, 196–7,
    225
  traditions 39, 99, 197
Christianity 2, 97, 153, 164. *See also*
    Jesus
  Constantine's adoption of 138
  core principle of 164
  and Emperor Julian 138
  and healing 37–45
  Protestant 172
  rise and role of plague 136
Christology 203–17
  and cancer 203–17
  and Henrietta Lacks 209–16
chronic/debilitating pain 71
Church 154–7
  and AIDS 154–7
  treatment that looks like 170–4
City Slickers 219
clergy
  burnout in 184–8
  and hospice chaplaincy 103
  and laity 136
  mission-driven focus of 188
code death 92

Cohn, Roy 158
"commendation" of death 98
"co-morbidities" of death 99
Cone, James 215
congregations 25–6
"constraint induced" movement 61
contagion. *See* faith and contagion
Copernicus 46, 53
Covid-19 pandemic 85, 97, 108, 131,
    134, 141, 146, 153, 185
cure 35–7

Danvers, Karina 160–1
"Dark Night" project 112
death
  bad 99
  code 92
  "commendation" of 98
  "co-morbidities" of 99
  good 94, 96, 98–100, 103–4
  mass 97, 137
  medicalized 92–6
*De humani corpora's Fabrica Libra
    septem* (Vesalius) 20
*Dialogue Concerning the Two Chief
    World Systems* (Galileo) 53
Dickens, Charles 99
disengagement 183–4, 187, 190
Donne, John
  *Hymn to God, My God, in My
    Sickness* 13–14
"Do No Harm" educational
    program 112
"dosage" 7
Dugdale, Lydia 90–2, 100–1
  Lost Art of Dying, The 100

emotional exhaustion 184
eudaimonia 196
evangelical Christians 169
evangelical Christian theologies 174
"everyday" medicine 4
existentialism 162

faith and contagion
   changes   132–5
   disease and disgust   139–41
   healing   37
   overview   131–2
   plague and religion   135–8
   and Ptolemaic cosmology   49–52
   relevance of past   145–6
   scapegoat prescription   141–5
"Faith that Heals, The" (Osler)   109
fast medicine   58–63
Father Damien of Molokai   9
Faulkner, William   145
first things   219
Flexner, Abraham   55, 57
Flexner model   55
flourishing   192–5
folk healer   36
forgiveness as health issue   178–81

Galen   46, 138
Galenic medicine   46–7, 49, 52, 54, 59
Galileo   53
   Dialogue Concerning the Two Chief World Systems   53
Gawande, Atul   95–6, 102
   Being Mortal   95
German placebo effect   79
Gerson, Jean   98
Gey, George Otto   203, 216–17
God's Hotel: A Doctor, a Hospital, and a Pilgrimage to the Heart of Medicine (Sweet)   58
good death   94, 96, 98–100, 103–4
Gould, Stephen Jay   6–7
Greene, Graham   183, 186
   Burnt Out Case, The   183, 186

Harvard Human Flourishing Program   179
Hauerwas, Stanley   72
healed by being seen   160–2
healers   27, 36, 57, 59

healing   4–5, 9–14, 220–2
   art of dying   96–102
   and Christianity   37–45
   divine power   44
   at the end   89–105
   faith   37
   by Jesus   38
   mechanics of   41
   medical   44, 72, 87, 213
   medicalized death   92–6
   physical   2, 6, 14, 23, 38–40, 84
   prayer as form of   84
   religious practice as form of   84
   times to die   90–2
health
   damage   176
   and forgiveness   178–81
health care
   power structure   158
   professionals   113
   providers   81
   proxy arrangements   97
   self-regulation in   87
   workers   94
Hebrew Bible   159
HeLa cells   204–7, 209, 212, 216–17
Hildegard of Bingen   58–62
   O Virtus Sapientiae   59
Hinduism   112
Hippocrates   48
Hippocratic tradition of medicine   46
HIV epidemic   149
   and America   157–60
   anxiety and acceptance   162–4
   case study   149–52
   and Churches   154–7
   healed by being seen   160–2
   worthy to be well   152–4
Homes, Oliver Wendell, Sr.   54–5
hopelessness   25, 62, 120
hospice care   103–4
human papillomavirus (HPV)   207
human violence   85

human well-being   73, 81, 116
"humoral" system   48
Hymn to God, My God, in My Sickness (Donne)   13–14

I and Thou (Buber)   163
idiosyncratic realism   20–1
I-it relationship   163
Imago Dei   164
immortality   203–17
    and cancer   203–17
Immortal Life of Henrietta Lacks, The (Skloot)   204, 206
immune response   77
implicit obligation   31
insurance policy   60, 97
integration   2–3, 23, 52, 54, 77, 103, 124–6, 195
interpersonal forgiveness   180
Ironson, Gail   112
Isenheim altarpiece   51
I-thou relationship   163

Jesus Christ   38–9, 41–3, 195, 210. *See also* Christianity
Johns Hopkins medical school   55–6

Koch, Robert   55
Koenig, Harold   110–11
Kushner, Tony   159–60

laboratory medicine   55, 205
Lacks, Henrietta
    Christology and   209–16
    in memory of her   216–17
    questions at the edge of medicine   207–9
    questions at the edge of theology   207–9
    theological resonance of   203–17
Lament for a Son (Wolterstorff)   86
Larson, David   109–11
last things   219, 225–8

Lazarus   44–5
Levin, Jeff   110
Levinas, Emmanuel   31–2
"Life Worth Living"   195
LinkedIn   185
logos   53
Lost Art of Dying, The (Dugdale)   100
Luhrman, Tanya   169
    When God Talks Back   169

Maslach, Christina   184
mass death   97, 137
McNeill, William Hardy   133, 137
    Plagues and Peoples   133
meaning effect   78–9, 82–4
medeor   5
medical anthropology   36
medical healing   44, 72, 87, 213
medicalized death   92–6
medical models   174–8
medical practice   164
medical technology   91, 226–7
medications   2, 60–2, 175–7
    cholesterol-lowering   107
    faith function as   107
    HIV   150–2
medicina   5
medicine   84–7
    changing modes of   52–8
    "everyday"   4
    fast   58–63
    language of   9–14
    ordinary   4
    Ptolemaic   45–9
    and Ptolemaic cosmology   49–52
    questions at the edge of   207–9
    and religion   1–3, 6–8
    vs. religion   8–9
    slow   58–63
medicus   5
mental health   7, 23, 68
    awareness of   186

diagnosis   169
  positive   120, 179
mind-body medicine   77
mindfulness meditation   113
Minow, Martha   180
  When Should Law Forgive?   180
miracles   35, 39, 42, 73–4, 77
  belief in   91
  religious patient   83
moral judgment   152
mortality   19–26
  healer   22–6
  idiosyncratic realism   20–1
  priest   22–6
  and sickness   24

naloxone   76
National Institute for Healthcare
    Research   110
neurological inability to feel pain   84
Nuland, Sherwin   94

obligation
  and calling   26–30
  and health care   29
  implicit   31
Oedipus (Sophocles)   140
ordinary medicine   4
ordinary religion   4
Osler, Sir William   55–6, 109
  "Faith that Heals, The"   109
Other
  as object   163
  objectified   162
  and self   163
  vulnerable   162
O Virtus Sapientiae (Hildegard of
    Bingen)   59

pain   85
  "alert" function of   84
  chronic/debilitating   71
  neurological inability to feel   84

phantom limb   71
  -related prayer   81
  spiritual   81 n.30
  vs. suffering   68–72
palliative care   103–5, 168, 193
phantom limb pain   71
Philosophical Investigations
    (Wittgenstein)   10
phlegm   48
physical healing   2, 6, 14, 23, 38–40,
    84
physical well-being   82
physicians   9, 29
  age of   35–7
  burnout in   184–8
  "geographical" knowledge   14
  human qualities   27
physiological self-modulation   77
placebo effect   76–80, 82–3
  German   79
placebos   73–6, 78, 113
  as generally an *external*
      treatment   77
  medical evidence for   77
  and prayer   76–80
  takes effect within patient   77
Plague, The (Camus)   140
Plagues and Peoples (McNeill)   133
prayers   73–6
  benefits of   77
  defined   80
  kind of   80–1
  in management of pain   80
  pain-related   81
  as part of spiritual immune
      system   77
  and placebo   76–80
  subjective recesses of   77
priests
  age of   35–7
  mortality   22–6
problem solvers   26–7
profession

cultural concept of 26
medical 26–7
Protestant Christianity 172
Ptolemaic cosmology 47, 49
and faith 49–52
and medicine 49–52
Ptolemaic medicine 45–9

questions at edge of medicine/
theology 207–9

randomized controlled trial
(RCT) 113–14, 114 n.23
religion 107–9
confounders 119–23
integration 124–6
language of 9–14
and medicine 1–3, 6–8
vs. medicine 8–9
ordinary 4
research 117–19
revolution in research on 109–12
webs of meaning 113–17
webs of truth 113–17
religious attitudes and practices 83
religious communities 97, 198
religious faith and communities 96
religious interventions 81
religious observance 125
religious participation 107, 111, 117, 120, 123
religious patient 83. *See also* caregiver
religious traditions and
communities 124
reorientations 24
responses to burnout 188–9
revitalization movements 137
Roman Catholic hospices and
hospitals 155
Rush, Benjamin 54

salvation 5, 8, 39, 68, 171, 173, 220, 226
salvus 5

Sartre, Jean Paul 162
Saunders, Cicely 103
scapegoat prescription 141–5
scripture 10, 30, 38–9, 43, 115, 125
Second World War 162
self-forgiveness 180
self-medication 77
self-modulations 77
Seventh Day Adventist Church 195
Skloot, Rebecca 204, 206, 217
*Immortal Life of Henrietta Lacks,
The* 204, 206
slow medicine 58–63
Smith, Bob 170
Snow, John 132
Sophocles
Oedipus 140
S.O.S. (Secular Organizations for
Sobriety) 172
spectrum healing 82–4
spiritual and religious orientations 77
spiritual crisis
burnout as 183–98
spiritual illness 5
spirituality 2, 4, 7, 38, 110, 117, 119–20, 155, 164
active 192
ascetic and world-denying
dimensions of 50
Christian 93
dimension of recovery 172
private 195
and theology 220
therapeutic role of 168
spiritual pain 81 n.30
Spiritual Well-Being scale 120
Stark, Rodney 137–8
stigma 152–3, 156, 175, 181. *See also*
HIV epidemic
Stone, John 11–13
Strichartz, Gary 67–8
suffering
vs. pain 68–72

Sweet, Victoria   60, 62
   God's Hotel: A Doctor, a Hospital, and a Pilgrimage to the Heart of Medicine   58

"talk therapy"   68
Taub, Edward   61
T-cell counts   156
telos of medicine   71
Terminator, The   225, 227
theological "proof of concept"   73
theological resonance of Henrietta Lacks   203–17
theology
   Christian   10, 86, 115, 196–7, 225
   questions at the edge of   207–9
therapy of hope and forgiveness   167–81
therapy of other agency   76–80
Thomas, Lewis   93–4
tikkun olam   5

Universal Fellowship of Metropolitan Community Churches (UFMCC)   154–5, 157

VanderWeele, Tyler   121–4
Vesalius, Andreas
   De humani corpora's Fabrica Libra septem   20
viriditas   59, 61–2
vital signs   7, 176, 220

Waiting for Godot (Beckett)   190
webs of meaning   113–17
webs of truth   113–17
"We Have AIDS" ecumenical Lenten worship service   156
Western monasticism   112
When God Talks Back (Luhrman)   169
When Should Law Forgive? (Minow)   180
Wilde, Oscar   99
Williams, Delores   214–15
Wilson, Bill   170
Winfrey, Oprah   204
Wittgenstein, Ludwig
   Philosophical Investigations   10
Wolterstorff, Nicholas   86
   Lament for a Son   86
work-life balance   194
worthy to be well   152–4

Yale Medical School   160
yellow bile   48